FUNDAMENTALS OF
SKELETAL
RADIOLOGY

Third Edition

Clyde A. Helms, MD
Professor of Radiology and Surgery
Department of Radiology
Duke University School of Medicine
Durham, North Carolina

ELSEVIER
SAUNDERS

**ELSEVIER
SAUNDERS**

The Curtis Center
170 S Independence Mall W 300E
Philadelphia, Pennsylvania 19106

FUNDAMENTALS OF SKELETAL RADIOLOGY, THIRD EDITION   ISBN 0-7216-0570-2
Copyright © 2005, Elsevier Inc. All rights reserved.

NOTICE

Radiology is an ever-changing field. Standard safety precautions must be followed, but as new
research and clinical experience broaden our knowledge, changes in treatment and drug therapy
may become necessary or appropriate. Readers are advised to check the most current product
information provided by the manufacturer of each drug to be administered to verify the
recommended dose, the method and duration of administration, and contraindications. It is the
responsibility of the licensed prescriber, relying on experience and knowledge of the patient, to
determine dosages and the best treatment for each individual patient. Neither the publisher nor the
author assumes any liability for any injury and/or damage to persons or property arising from this
publication.

Previous editions copyrighted 1989, 1995

International Standard Book Number 0-7216-0570-2

Acquisitions Editor: Allan Ross
Developmental Editor: Edward Pontee
Publishing Services Manager: Melissa Lastarria
Senior Designer: Kathi Gosche

Printed in the United States of America

Last digit is the print number: 9 8 7 6 5 4 3 2 1

FUNDAMENTALS OF
SKELETAL
RADIOLOGY

Mike Mackenzie

01706   341100

A/E   X-RAY   HOPE HOSP.

This book is dedicated to

Jason

Benjamin

and

Austin.

Like medical students and residents they love to learn

and are a joy to teach.

Foreword to the Second Edition

Clyde Helms, as a radiologist in training during the mid 70s, was, in many ways, the ideal radiology resident. Able, perceptive, informed, and responsible, he progressed through the various stages of residency training in superb fashion. On the other hand, he was different. Whereas the traditional "best resident" always had at hand exhaustive lists of differential diagnoses, Dr. Helms quietly ignored the trivial, the esoteric, and the information that was not likely to serve him in his work as a radiologist in the "real world," sometimes to the discomfiture of the radiology faculty of the University of California, San Francisco (of which I was then a junior member). Whereas the traditional "best resident" was suitably in awe of the faculty (many of whom were truly awesome), Dr. Helms fearlessly challenged what he perceived as unsupportable dogma. Not one to sit still for pretension, he poked gentle (and sometimes not so gentle) fun at the faculty. Occasional pranks were perpetrated, sometimes at the expense of members of the faculty. No one was immune, no matter how lofty his status. Dr. Helms, as the Sinatra song goes, did it his way. Irreverent, witty, occasionally outrageous, and a superb radiologist, he completed his residency and went on to fulfill his military commitment.

He returned to UCSF 3 years later as a faculty member in the skeletal radiology section. That he had not changed was immediately apparent. Faculty meetings are disrupted by his irreverent remarks, frequently hilarious. Now a mentor, his teaching reflects the same realistic, nontraditional approach he used as a resident. He emphasizes not the exotic or esoteric but the practical, the information that is critical in the day-to-day practice of radiology. Incorporated into his teaching method are mnemonics, one or two of which might not be recommended for family viewing. On the other hand, if they work, why not use them? An increasingly large number of young radiologists (his residents and former residents) will attest that, indeed, they do work. The teaching may be unorthodox, but the learning is real and substantial.

This volume is also unorthodox. Several excellent, superbly researched and crafted treatises on skeletal radiology are available to the radiology resident and practicing radiologist. This volume is not intended as an exhaustive compendium of skeletal radiology. Rather it is, as indicated by the title, an exposition of the *basics* of skeletal radiology. In keeping with his personalized, unusual approach to teaching, he begins with a discussion of radiologic examinations that should *not* be performed. The remainder of the book deals with skeletal conditions that radiologists are likely to encounter any day of the week. The reader who wishes to become familiar with Scheie syndrome or tricho-rhinophalangeal dysplasia Type II must look elsewhere.

Rather than the usual, formal language found in other radiology texts, the reader will encounter the vernacular used by all radiologists when they discuss their work with other radiologists. The text is much like Dr. Helms himself—witty, irreverent, unpretentious, and fast-paced. The reader will find the book refreshing, eminently readable, and highly informative.

The ideal condition
Would be, I admit, that men should be right by instinct;
But since we are all likely to go astray,
The reasonable thing is to learn from those who can teach.
Sophocles

Clyde Helms can teach!

Hideyo Minagi, M.D.

Foreword

I consider the opportunity to write the forward to this book an honor. I have had the opportunity to work alongside of Clyde Helms for a number of years. During his career as an outstanding musculoskeletal radiologist, he has trained numerous residents and fellows, has educated orthopedic residents and surgeons, and influenced emergency department physicians, as well as physician's assistants. Clyde has changed many a career path for medical students by showing them how much fun the specialty of radiology can be. Radiology residents have chosen musculoskeletal fellowships to be in his tutelage for an additional year of their training. I know. I was one of those residents.

The individuals that have been affected by Clyde will all agree about one thing. Clyde can teach, and he can have fun while doing it. It is one thing, however, to be a good teacher, another to be able to put it into words. Clyde's *Fundamentals of Skeletal Radiology* is so successful because he gives you a glimpse into his ability to communicate and share his teaching style with the reader. It is, as he says, "informal and casual." It is easy to read, filled with facts, and entertaining as well. This book is a reflection of Clyde Helms, full of facts, but not full of himself.

Nancy M. Major, MD
Associate Professor Radiology and Surgery
Division of Musculoskeletal Imaging
Duke University Medical Center
Durham, NC

Preface

The third edition of this book shows little substantial change from the second; however, it has refinements and subtle corrections that make it a more accurate reflection of my experience as a bone radiologist for the past nearly 30 years. The chapters on MRI have been considerably updated to reflect the ongoing improvements in that area.

In keeping with the previous editions and my basic personality I have kept the style of writing very informal and casual. When the first edition was written I was concerned that my peers and mentors would have judged me to be too irreverent and superficial in dealing with a very serious and weighty subject. To my surprise the first edition was well received and became quite popular. I'm sure many did think it was irreverent and superficial, but now, fifteen years later, those criticisms wouldn't bother me. In fact, this book *is* irreverent and superficial! It's meant to be. It's not meant to be disrespectful to a profession that is worthy of the highest respect – it's merely a style of teaching that makes learning easier for many of us. Once the basics of a subject are mastered one can delve more deeply into a topic. Other books have been written to address that aspect of bone radiology. Use this book to get started and to have some fun while you learn.

Clyde A. Helms

Contents

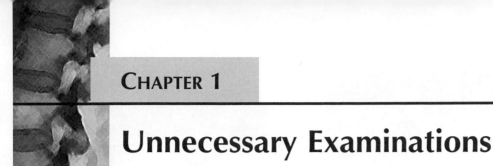

CHAPTER 1

Unnecessary Examinations

Before beginning to learn how to interpret pathologic skeletal films, it is important to briefly consider unnecessary skeletal radiographic examinations. Dr. Ferris Hall from Boston first brought to my attention the idea that just because we *could* x-ray something didn't mean that we *should*. His article entitled "Overutilization of Radiologic Examinations," which was published in the August 1976 issue of *Radiology,*[1] details many examples of overuse and misuse of radiologic examinations. This article, even though it is more than 25 years old, and a similar article by Dr. Herbert Abrams, which was published in the *New England Journal of Medicine,*[2] should be mandatory reading for every intern before he or she begins to order examinations.

There are many reasons why it is undesirable to have unnecessary radiologic examinations, including excess cost, excess radiation, waste of patient's time, waste of technician's and radiologist's time, false hopes and expectations based on the outcome of the examination, and, not least of all, they indicate a breakdown in the logical thought pattern concerning the patient's workup.

Many examinations are ordered because of so-called medicolegal considerations. It is believed that if a certain finding is not documented (e.g., a broken rib), the doctor could be sued. In fact, few, if any, examples of medicolegal "covering yourself" types of examinations are valid. With the move toward greater consumer awareness, lawsuits in the future are more likely to result from unnecessary radiation exposure because of needless examinations rather than from too few examinations.

EXAMPLES OF UNNECESSARY EXAMINATIONS

Skull Series. Except for a depressed skull fracture or the presence of intracranial metallic fragments, there is no reason to order a skull series for trauma. This is one of the most abused examinations

in radiology, costing millions of dollars per year unnecessarily. There is virtually no finding on a skull series that will alter the next step in the patient's workup. Presence or absence of a fracture should not influence whether the patient receives a computed tomography (CT) scan or a magnetic resonance imaging (MRI) examination. A CT scan or MRI examination is obtained for other reasons: continued unconsciousness or focal neurologic signs. The plain films only delay the eventual diagnosis, and in a patient with a subdural or an epidural hematoma, that delay could be fatal.[3] The mortality from intracranial bleeds is significantly increased as the time to surgical decompression is increased; therefore, any delay caused by obtaining unnecessary examinations (skull films) is potentially harmful. There are no findings on a plain skull series to indicate (or not indicate) subdural or epidural hematoma (Fig. 1-1). Less than 10% of patients with fractures have subdural or epidural hematomas, and up to 60% of patients with subdural or epidural bleeds have no fractures.[4] Therefore, why order the examinations? Medicolegal reasons? On the contrary! It is well documented that delays in diagnosis in this setting can be fatal; therefore, ordering unnecessary examinations might in fact be asking for a lawsuit! The American College of Radiology has published appropriateness criteria for when to order particular examinations and has endorsed head CT scanning as the initial study of choice in trauma.[5]

In spite of much documentation in the radiology and emergency room (ER) literature showing the lack of utility of skull films in trauma, they continue to be routinely ordered in many ERs throughout North America. A survey performed in 1991 by Hackney and published in *Radiology*[6] showed that more than 50% of the hospitals in the study "often or always" obtained skull films for trauma. Every hospital had CT scanning available. What are they thinking? Obviously, they are not thinking about what a skull film will show them

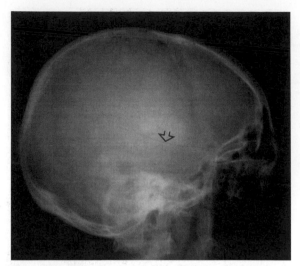

FIGURE 1-1 Skull fracture. A thin radiolucent line characteristic of a skull fracture is noted *(arrow)* extending obliquely across the temporal bone. A fracture in this area is often associated with an epidural hematoma because the middle meningeal artery lies here. This finding by itself, however, has little or no significance and must be correlated with clinical findings.

FIGURE 1-2 Waters' view of the sinuses. This film is obtained with the patient's head slightly tilted upward (as if he or she were drinking water—apologies to Dr. Waters). It is an excellent film to obtain when the maxillary sinuses need to be seen. When it is done with the patient in an upright position, air-fluid levels can be seen *(arrow)*.

that might affect their treatment, because it won't change a thing whether it's positive or negative.

Sinus Series. It is true that an opaque sinus and/or an air-fluid level can be seen with sinusitis. But often the patient with these findings is asymptomatic, and just as often in another patient the sinus series is interpreted as normal when the patient has typical clinical findings of sinusitis. Both of these patients are treated on the basis of their clinical, not radiographic, presentation, which is appropriate. Therefore, the information from the sinus series is ignored. If this is the way you practice—and many recommend that as being proper—don't order the sinus series, treat the patient. Reserve the sinus series for the patient who doesn't respond to treatment or has an unusual presentation. Also, if it is only sinusitis that concerns you, most times a simple upright Waters' view (Fig. 1-2) to examine the maxillary and frontal sinuses, rather than a full sinus series, will suffice, saving money and decreasing patient exposure.[7]

Nasal Bone. A nasal series is often requested to see if a patient has suffered a broken nose after trauma to the face. So what if the nasal bone is fractured? It won't be cast. It won't be reduced. In other words, no treatment will be given regardless of what the x-ray shows. Therefore, don't order the films in the first place. Occasionally, a nasal bone is badly enough displaced to warrant intervention, but even then an acute, posttraumatic

x-ray adds nothing for the patient except expense and radiation exposure. A facial series or a CT scan to search for additional fractures might be in order, but not a nasal series.

Rib Series. Fractured ribs are commonly seen in any radiologic practice. The significance of the finding of a fractured rib or ribs is not well appreciated by most physicians. If the truth be known, the finding of a rib fracture after trauma has almost no clinical significance and does not alter treatment. One must rule out a pneumothorax and even a lung contusion, both of which are uncommon and are best done on chest films, not a rib series. In older patients with chest wall pain and rib fractures from undetermined causes, it is extremely difficult and often impossible to differentiate a pathologic rib fracture through a metastatic focus from a posttraumatic rib fracture. Hence, x-raying a patient with focal rib pain to find a fracture serves little purpose other than finding a cause for the pain. Most rib series can be eliminated without changing the way the patient is treated.

Coccyx. Although it is not a common x-ray examination, there are occasionally requests to x-ray the coccyx to rule out a fracture. As with the nasal bone and ribs, a fracture in this location will not be cast or reduced. Also, this examination has a significantly greater gonadal radiation dose than a rib or nasal series. Because no treatment is predicated on the x-ray results, don't order the x-ray for routine trauma to the coccyx.

Lumbar Spine. Plain films of the lumbar spine are probably the most abused examinations in radiology. They give the greatest gonadal radiation dose of any plain film examination, and, in most cases, they offer no diagnostic information that will be acted on by the physician. A significant number of lumbar spine films are done in a population younger than 40 years who have acute onset of back pain after lifting or straining. There is virtually no plain film x-ray finding in this patient subgroup that can be responsible for the acute problem or that can be treated. Even the severest spondylolisthesis cannot unequivocally be said to be the origin of the symptoms. Disc herniation cannot be identified. Tumors and infections are not clinical considerations in this setting. Treatment invariably consists of rest, nonsteroidal anti-inflammatory drugs (NSAIDs), generally relaxing the muscle groups, and then flexion and extension exercises to strengthen the muscles. Radiographs have nothing to offer unless the pain is atypical or the clinical picture is clouded by other considerations (such as intravenous drug use, in which case infection must be ruled out).

The gonadal radiation dose from a lumbar spine film is the same as that from a daily chest x-ray for 6,[8] 16,[9] or 98 years,[10] depending on which study you choose to believe. These studies were based on a three-view lumbosacral spine series and do not include the oblique views routinely obtained in many practices. Subtle osseous changes found on oblique views are thought by many orthopedists to be insignificant in most cases anyway.

So when should a lumbosacral spine series be ordered? It should be ordered in cases of severe trauma, possible primary or metastatic tumor, and possible infection. Acute low back pain with radicular signs is not an indication for a spine series. An MRI examination will show disc herniation and would be the preferred examination compared with plain films, if clinically warranted. Generally, a lumbar spine MRI examination is performed only after a failed course of conservative therapy if disc disease is clinically suspected.

Metabolic Bone Survey. Many institutions routinely order metabolic bone surveys in patients with hyperparathyroidism or renal osteodystrophy to look for Looser's zone fractures, brown tumors, and subperiosteal bone resorption. Most institutions have replaced the bone survey with hand films, which is preferable in regard to patient expense and radiation dose. Subperiosteal bone resorption is seen earliest and easiest on the middle phalanges, radial sides (Fig. 1-3), and is virtually pathognomonic for hyperparathyroidism. Looser's zone fractures are rare and are not treated anyway. Brown tumors are uncommon and also are not treated. Therefore, if no treatment is based on

FIGURE 1-3 **Phalanges with subperiosteal bone resorption.** Subperiosteal bone resorption is seen as a subtle irregularity or interruption of the cortex. It is best seen on the radial aspect of the middle phalanges (*arrows*) and is pathognomonic for hyperparathyroidism.

the x-ray findings, the survey only satisfies curiosity and is not worth the patient's money or radiation exposure.

Metastatic Bone Survey. Little useful information is obtained from the majority of metastatic bone surveys. Occult lesions that are not found on radionuclide bone scans are seldom encountered. Radionuclide scans are more effective at picking up most metastatic lesions and could be substituted for bone surveys with less cost and better diagnostic yield.[11] Many investigators believe that searching for bone metastases is not warranted in every patient with a primary tumor unless finding metastatic disease (mets) will obviate surgery or otherwise change the patient's therapy. Radionuclide bone scans with x-rays of questionable or clinically suspicious areas make more sense than a complete metastatic bone survey. An exception to this is in patients with multiple myeloma. Radionuclide bone scans are often negative in multiple myeloma even with marked skeletal involvement; hence, a plain film bone survey is warranted in these patients.

Ankle Series. The primary cause for presentation to ERs in North America is an ankle sprain, with more than 30,000 ankle sprains per day reported.[12] Ligamentous injuries can easily be clinically differentiated from significant fractures. One study showed a 50% reduction of ankle films with no fractures missed when the radiology resident simply examined the patient.[13] Another study revealed that if the patient were able to walk three steps immediately after the injury or during the examination in the ER, there was almost zero chance of a fracture.[14] This study was one of several to use what has been called the "Ottawa Rules" for when to obtain ankle x-rays. They are so-named after the hometown of the first authors to implement them and are in widespread use today in the majority of ERs in North America. Small bony avulsions receive the same treatment as ligament tears and are often difficult to differentiate from accessory ossicles (Fig. 1-4). Therefore, in most cases, the x-ray is not a factor in determining the patient's treatment and should be skipped.

Lumbar Myelograms. One of the most painful radiologic examinations extant is the lumbar myelogram, in which a spinal needle is placed into the subarachnoid space of the lumbar spine and contrast material is injected (Fig. 1-5). Although this is done for tumors, it is most commonly performed in the workup of lumbar disc disease. Many stud-

FIGURE 1-5 **Lumbar myelogram.** An iodinated contrast material has been injected into the subarachnoid space by way of a spinal needle. A large extradural defect is seen that is caused by a disc protrusion. A tumor could have a similar appearance. This examination can be quite painful, has occasional long-lasting complications, and gives no information that could not be obtained with an MRI examination. In some institutions, it requires an overnight stay in the hospital as well. For these reasons the standard of practice today is an MRI examination.

FIGURE 1-4 **Ankle after trauma.** Calcific densities around the ankle that can be mistaken for avulsions are often seen (*arrow*). When rounded and smoothly corticated, as in this example, they are either accessory ossicles or old avulsions. An acute avulsion is best diagnosed clinically by noting point tenderness at ligament insertion sites. Because a ligament can avulse with or without a fragment of bone being attached, the x-ray finding will not influence the patient's treatment.

ies show that CT scanning or MRI of the lumbar spine is more accurate than myelography in diagnosing disc disease, and these studies emphasize that CT or MRI should be the study of choice. Many surgeons, however, still request myelograms in addition to the CT or MRI examination, when only the CT or MRI examination need be performed. In addition to being painful, the myelogram produces side effects in some people that can be pronounced and debilitating; the myelogram occasionally necessitates overnight hospitalization; the radiation dose from the myelogram is greater overall than with CT; and perhaps most important, the myelogram is not as accurate and does not give as complete a picture of additional back structures as the CT or MRI examination (Fig. 1-6). We can hope that the myelogram will go the way of the pneumoencephalogram and the epidural venogram.

So far as choosing between CT scanning and MRI of the lumbar spine for disc disease and

FIGURE 1-6 **Lumbar MRI.** Axial T1-weighted (*top*) and T2-weighted (*bottom*) images through the L4-5 disc space show a focal lateral disc protrusion (*arrows*) that is encroaching on the left neuroforamen. This type of disc protrusion would likely not be seen with a myelogram.

spinal stenosis, an MRI examination will give much more diagnostic information and is considered the state-of-the-art imaging examination for the spine.

Cervical Spine. Many ERs routinely order cervical spine (C-spine) films on all trauma patients, primarily because of the horrible consequences of not stabilizing a fractured neck. This is ridiculous. It has been demonstrated in numerous publications that patients who are alert and have no C-spine pain have almost zero chance of having a fracture.[15] If the patient is unconscious, obtunded for whatever reason, not able to communicate, or has a significant fracture elsewhere, all bets are off. But if the patient is alert and has no pain with motion on clinical examination of the neck, no posterior midline tenderness, and no neurologic deficits, no C-spine film need be performed.[16]

TECHNICAL CONSIDERATIONS

Avoiding unnecessary examinations constitutes only one way to decrease unnecessary radiation exposure in the general population. Another way to significantly diminish exposure is to collimate the x-ray beam tighter. One study reported that if collimation were limited just to the size of the film,

radiation dose could be reduced by one third.[17] Exposure could be further reduced by having proper filtration, fast screen–film combination, and adequate gonadal shielding. Digital radiography, which is gaining widespread use, will further help to decrease radiation dose. Certainly having properly trained technicians and properly functioning equipment will diminish the number of retakes. These should be high-priority goals for all radiologists to make our specialty more cost-effective and to provide better service to both the referring clinician and the patient. It should be part of every radiologist's responsibility to help educate and guide the unknowing clinician in obtaining the appropriate imaging examinations and eliminating those that are unnecessary.

REFERENCES

1. Hall F: Overutilization of radiological examinations. Radiology 1976;120:443-448.
2. Abrams HL: The "overutilization" of x-rays: Sounding board. N Engl J Med 1979;300:1213-1216.
3. Seelig JM, Becker DP, Miller JD, et al: Traumatic acute subdural hematoma. N Engl J Med 1981;304:1511-1518.
4. Masters JS, McClean PM, Arcarese JS, et al: Skull x-ray examinations after head trauma. N Engl J Med 1987;316:84-91.
5. American College of Radiology. ACR Appropriateness Criteria Head Trauma. 2001. Available at http://www.acr.org, accessed July 29, 2004.
6. Hackney DB: Skull radiography in the evaluation of acute head trauma: A survey of current practice. Radiology 1991;181:711-714.
7. Williams JJ, Roberts L, Distell B, Simel D: Diagnosing sinusitis by x-ray: Comparing a single Waters view to 4-view paranasal sinus radiographs. J Gen Intern Med 1992;7:481-485.
8. Webster EW, Merrill OE: Radiation hazards: II. Measurements of gonadal dose in radiologic examinations. N Engl J Med 1957;257:811-819.
9. Antoku S, Russell WJ: Dose to the active bone marrow, gonads, and skin from roentgenography and flouroscopy. Radiology 1957;101:669-678.
10. Andron GM, Crooks HE: Gonad radiation dose from diagnostic procedures. Br J Radiol 1957;30:295-297.
11. Mall JC, Bekerman C, Hoffer PB, et al: A unified radiological approach to the detection of skeletal metastases. Radiology 1976;118:323-329.
12. Cheung Y, Rosenberg ZS: MR imaging of ligamentous abnormalities of the ankle and foot. Magn Reson Imaging Clin N Am 2001;9:507-531.
13. Auletta A, Conway W, Hayes C, et al: Indications for radiography in patients with acute ankle injuries: Role of the physical examination. Am J Roentgenol 1991;157:789-791.
14. Stiell I, Greenberg G, McKnight R, et al: Decision rules for the use of radiography in acute ankle injuries. JAMA 1993;269:1127-1132.

15. Mirvis S, Diaconis J, Chirico P, et al: Protocol-driven radiologic evaluation of suspected cervical spine injury: Efficacy study. Radiology 1989;170:831-834.
16. Hoffman JR, Mower WR, Wolfson AB, et al: Validity of a set of clinical criteria to rule out injury to the cervical spine in patients with blunt trauma. N Engl J Med 2000;343:94-99.

17. Morgan RH: Hearings before the Committee on Commerce, Science and Transportation. U.S. Senate, an oversight of radiation health and safety. 95th Congress, 1st session, June 1977, pp. 241-266.

CHAPTER 2

Benign Lytic Lesions

A benign, bubbly lytic lesion of bone is probably one of the most common skeletal findings a radiologist encounters. The differential diagnosis can be quite lengthy and is usually given on an "Aunt Minnie" basis (I know that's Aunt Minnie because she *looks* like Aunt Minnie); in other words, the differential diagnosis is structured on how the lesion looks to the radiologist, using his or her experience as a guide. This method, called *"pattern identification,"* certainly has merit, but it can lead to many erroneous conclusions if not tempered with some logic. For instance, most radiologists would justifiably miss the diagnosis of a rare presentation of a primary malignant neoplasm that initially looks benign. Many of these radiologists would subsequently insist on including primary malignant neoplasms in their benign lytic differential even though the rare malignancy is "one in a million." If every differential is geared to cover even the long shots, there would be a lot of extremely long differentials, and the clinicians wouldn't get much useful information from us. We may as well give the clinician the index to a multivolume bone book as give a differential that will never miss anything.

Then again, you don't want a differential diagnosis list that is wrong half of the time. You could almost do better with a coin flip. I'm willing to accept a differential that is accurate (that is, one that contains the correct diagnosis) 95% of the time. This is acceptable to me for most skeletal entities; however, I would be remiss if I were willing to accept a 1-out-of-20 miss rate for fractures and dislocations. Nevertheless, for most of the entities in this book I will accept a 95% accuracy differential and would expect most radiologists to concur. If you want to be more accurate than that, you simply add more diagnoses to the list of differential possibilities.

The shorter the differential diagnosis list, the easier it is to remember and apply. As the differential list gets longer, it generally gets more accurate, but it can be difficult to remember and often falls into disuse. Mnemonics are helpful in recalling long lists of information, and I will pass on many that I use; many people, however, do not like to use mnemonics (for no good reason that I've been able to ascertain) and will just have to use whatever method works for them to remember the differentials. The list of entities that cause benign lytic lesions is quite long, therefore a mnemonic is helpful in recalling them.

I was a flight surgeon in the Air Force before my radiology residency, and I would spend a half day a week or so with the radiologist, trying to pick up some pearls. This radiologist was Ivan Barrett, and he did me a great favor. He taught me the mnemonic FEGNOMASHIC, which is made up from the first letter of each of the entities in the differential of benign lytic lesions of bone. The F stands for fibrous dysplasia, the E for enchondroma, and so on, as I will show. I diligently learned what each letter stood for, even though I had no idea what most of the processes were or looked like on an x-ray. Before I could learn another mnemonic from Ivan (I was a slow learner), I moved away to begin my residency.

Sure enough, the first week of residency, in a formal conference with 15 to 20 residents present, I was chosen as the sacrificial lamb among the first-year residents to take an unknown case. It happened to be a benign lytic lesion, which I proceeded to expound on with a list of 12 to 15 differential possibilities. The conference room got quiet, I was thanked cordially but a little frostily, and the conference was adjourned. One of the first-year residents, who I barely knew at the time, asked how I knew so many of the possibilities on that case, because the staff member showing the case (who was a chest radiologist) didn't even know that many. I explained, with a straight face, that those just seemed like the logical things to mention. I was trying to be matter of fact and not come off as too much of a show-off, but I couldn't help laughing. I then told the resident how I had learned a single mnemonic, and how by luck it made me seem to know a lot more than I really did. He and the rest of my fellow residents were relieved that I really wasn't any smarter or more advanced than they were, and quickly learned the mnemonic themselves. I became hopelessly addicted to mnemonics from that day on.

FEGNOMASHIC

FEGNOMASHIC is defined in *"Funk and Wagner's" Unabridged Dictionary, 13th edition,* as "one who uses mnemonics." It serves as a nice starting point for discussing possibilities that appear as benign lytic lesions in bone. That mnemonic has been in general use for many years, but I have never heard a claim as to who first coined it. The first mention of it that I saw in print was in 1972, in a radiology article by Gold and colleagues.[1] By itself, it is merely a long list—about 14 entities—and needs to be coupled with other criteria to shorten the list into a manageable form for each particular case. For instance, if the lesion is epiphyseal, only three to five entities, depending on how accurate you care to be, need to be mentioned. If multiple lesions are present, only half a dozen entities need to be discussed. Ways of narrowing the differential are discussed later in this chapter.

The next step after learning the names of all the lesions is getting some idea of what each one looks like. This is where experience becomes a factor. For the medical student or first-year resident it's difficult to go beyond saying that they all look lytic or bubbly and benign. However, the fourth-year resident should have no trouble differentiating between a unicameral bone cyst and a giant cell tumor (GCT), because he or she has seen examples of each many times before and knows what each looks like. The fourth-year resident may have a hard time verbalizing the differences but should be able to tell them apart.

A novice can quickly gain experience by looking at the examples of each of these lesions in a major skeletal radiology textbook. In fact, I highly recommend that you compare my description and differential points on each lesion with multiple examples in other books. Some of these lesions can only be diagnosed radiologically on a "pattern identification" or "Aunt Minnie" basis. In other words, there are no hard and fast criteria to differentiate some lesions from others.

After getting a feel for what each lesion looks like radiographically, and overcoming the frustration that builds when you realize that many of them look alike, you should try to learn ways to differentiate each lesion from the others. I have developed a number of keys that I call *"discriminators"* that will help to differentiate each lesion. These discriminators are 90 to 95% accurate (I will mention when they are more or less accurate, in my experience) and are by no means meant to be absolutes or dogma. They are guidelines, but they have a high confidence rate.

Textbooks rarely tell you that a finding "always" or "never" occurs. They temper their descriptions with "virtually always," "usually," or "characteristically." I have tried to pick out findings that come as close to "always" as I can, realizing that I will only be 95% accurate. That's good enough for me. If it's not good enough for you, you will need to get your own differential criteria or discriminators. Try these and see if they work for you. If they don't work, modify them as necessary. But whatever you do, develop *reasons* for including things in your differential. Have concrete criteria of some kind for including or excluding each entity.

Following are brief descriptions of each entity, as complete descriptions are readily available in any skeletal radiology textbook. What I dwell on, however, are the points that are unique for each entity, thereby enabling differentiation from the others. Table 2-1 is a synopsis of these discriminators.

FIBROUS DYSPLASIA

It is unfortunate that this differential starts with fibrous dysplasia, because fibrous dysplasia can look like almost anything. It can be wild-looking, a discrete lucency, patchy, sclerotic, expansile, multiple, and a host of other descriptions. It is, therefore, difficult to look at a bubbly lytic lesion and unequivocally say it is or is not fibrous dysplasia. When assessing such a lesion, radiology residents usually say, "I suppose it *could* be fibrous dysplasia, but I'm not sure." The resident is feeling insecure and becomes defensive right off, setting the tone for the entire differential diagnosis. It would be better if the differential started on a positive note, for example, with GCT or chondroblastoma, for which there are some hard and definite criteria. That way the resident would set a tone of self-assurance and decisiveness rather than appear wishy-washy. Then, when mentioning fibrous dysplasia and using the same words, "I suppose it *could* be fibrous dysplasia, but I'm not sure," he or she is looked on as showing thoughtful deliberation rather than insecurity or ignorance. It's pure gamesmanship, but it makes a difference in how the resident is perceived.

How do you know whether to include or exclude fibrous dysplasia if it can look like almost anything? Experience is the best guideline. In other words, look in a few textbooks and find as

TABLE 2-1   Differential Criteria for Benign Lytic Bone Lesions Mnemonic: FEGNOMASHIC

F	*Fibrous dysplasia:* No pain or periosteal reaction; if in tibia, mention adamantinoma
E	*Enchondroma:* Must have calcification, except in phalanges; no pain or periostitis
	Eosinophilic granuloma (EG): Must be younger than 30 years
G	*Giant cell tumor (GCT):* (1) Epiphyses must be closed; (2) must be epiphyseal *and* abut the articular surface; (3) eccentric; (4) well-defined but nonsclerotic border
N	*Nonossifying fibroma (NOF):* Must be younger than 30 years; no pain or periostitis
O	*Osteoblastoma:* Mentioned whenever ABC is mentioned, even if patient is older than 30 years
M	*Metastatic disease (mets) and myeloma:* Must be older than 40 years
A	*Aneurysmal bone cyst (ABC):* Must be younger than 30 years; expansile
S	*Solitary bone cyst:* Must be centrally located; younger than 30 years; no pain or periostitis
H	*Hyperparathyroidism (Brown tumor):* Must have other evidence of hyperparathyroidism
I	*Infection:* If adjacent to a joint, must involve the joint (weak)
C	*Chondroblastoma:* Must be younger than 30 years; epiphyseal
	Chondromyxoid fibroma: Mention when considering nonossifying fibroma

Younger Than 30 Years	No Periostitis or Pain	Epiphyseal	Multiple
EG	Fibrous dysplasia	Chondroblastoma	(Mnemonic: FEEMHI)
ABC	Enchondroma	Infection	Fibrous dysplasia
NOF	NOF	GCT	EG
Chondroblastoma	Solitary bone cyst	Geode	Enchondroma
Solitary bone cyst		(EG and ABC are optional)	Mets and Myeloma
			Hyperparathyroidism
			Infection

many different examples as you can; get a feeling for what fibrous dysplasia looks like. A few examples are shown here (Figs. 2-1 to 2-6), but poring over another textbook for 10 to 15 minutes will be time well spent.

Fibrous dysplasia will not have periostitis associated with it; therefore, if periostitis is present, you can safely exclude fibrous dysplasia. It would be possible to have a pathologic fracture through an area of fibrous dysplasia, which then had periostitis, but I have never seen this occur. Fibrous dysplasia virtually never undergoes malignant degeneration, and should not be a painful lesion in the long bones unless there is a fracture.

Fibrous dysplasia can be either monostotic (most commonly) or polyostotic, and has a predilection for the pelvis, proximal femur, ribs, and skull. When it is present in the pelvis, it is invariably present in the ipsilateral proximal femur (see Figs. 2-3 and 2-4). I have seen only one case in which the pelvis was involved with fibrous dysplasia and the proximal femur was spared. The proximal femur, however, may be affected alone, without involvement in the pelvis (see Figs. 2-5 and 2-6).

The classic description of fibrous dysplasia is that it has a ground-glass or smoky appearing matrix. This description confuses people rather than helps them, and I do not recommend using "ground-glass appearance" as a buzz word for fibrous dysplasia. Fibrous dysplasia is often purely lytic and becomes hazy or takes on a ground-glass

look as the matrix calcifies. It can go on to calcify quite a bit, and then it presents as a sclerotic lesion. Also, I often see other lytic lesions that have a distinct ground-glass appearance; therefore, the ground-glass quality can be misleading.

When a lesion in the tibia that has fibrous dysplasia in the differential diagnosis is encountered, an adamantinoma should also be mentioned (Fig. 2-7). An adamantinoma is a malignant tumor that radiographically and histologically resembles fibrous dysplasia. It occurs almost exclusively in the tibia and the jaw (for unknown reasons) and is rare. Because it is rare, you may choose not to include it in your memory bank—you won't miss more than one or two in your lifetime, even if you are a busy radiologist.

Polyostotic fibrous dysplasia occasionally occurs in association with café au lait spots on the skin (dark-pigmented, freckle-like lesions) and precocious puberty. This complex is called McCune-Albright syndrome. The bony lesions in this syndrome, and even in the simple polyostotic form, often occur unilaterally (that is, in one half of the body). This doesn't happen often enough to be of any diagnostic use in differentiating fibrous dysplasia from other lesions. The presence of multiple lesions in the jaw has been termed cherubism, which relates to the physical appearance of the affected child. Such children present with puffed out cheeks, producing an "angelic" look. The jaw lesions in cherubism regress in adulthood.

FIGURE 2-2 **Fibrous dysplasia.** The ribs often are involved with fibrous dysplasia, as in this example. When the posterior ribs are involved, the process often is a lytic expansile lesion, whereas when the anterior ribs are involved, it is commonly a sclerotic process.

FIGURE 2-1 **Fibrous dysplasia.** A predominantly lytic lesion with some sclerosis and expansion is seen in the distal half of the radius in a child. A long lesion in a long bone typifies fibrous dysplasia. Although parts of this lesion indeed have a ground-glass appearance, most of it does not. Expansion and bone deformity such as this are commonly seen in fibrous dysplasia.

Fibrous dysplasia often has areas of chondroid matrix, which, when biopsied, can resemble chondrosarcoma (as can any chondral tissue). I have seen sampling errors result in inappropriate radical surgery when the diagnosis should have been made on the plain films with no biopsy performed.

Discriminator: No periosteal reaction is present.

ENCHONDROMA AND EOSINOPHILIC GRANULOMA

Enchondroma

The most common benign cystic lesion of the phalanges is an enchondroma (Fig. 2-8). Enchondromas occur in any bone formed from cartilage and may be central, eccentric, expansile, or nonexpansile. They

FIGURE 2-3 **Fibrous dysplasia.** An expansile mixed lytic/sclerotic process in the proximal femur is a common pattern for fibrous dysplasia. Note that the supra-acetabular region also is involved. The ipsilateral proximal femur is invariably affected when the pelvis is involved with fibrous dysplasia.

FIGURE 2-4 **Fibrous dysplasia.** The entire pelvis and proximal femurs are diffusely involved with polyostotic fibrous dysplasia. The pelvis is severely deformed with predominantly lytic lesions. The proximal femurs are involved with both lytic and sclerotic lesions.

FIGURE 2-6 **Monostotic fibrous dysplasia.** Another example of proximal femur involvement that shows a lytic lesion with a thick sclerotic border reminiscent of a chronic infection. This is characteristic of fibrous dysplasia in the hip.

FIGURE 2-5 **Monostotic fibrous dysplasia.** The proximal femur is a common place for monostotic fibrous dysplasia. This presentation is typical and should not be confused with an infection. Some speckled calcification is noted within the lesion that should not be misconstrued as chondroid calcification in an enchondroma.

invariably contain calcified chondroid matrix (Fig. 2-9*A*), except when in the phalanges. If a cystic lesion is present without calcified chondroid matrix anywhere except in the phalanges, I will not include enchondroma in my differential.

Often it is difficult to differentiate between an enchondroma and a bone infarct. Although some of the following criteria are helpful in separating an infarct from an enchondroma, they are not foolproof. An infarct usually has a well-defined, densely sclerotic, serpiginous border, whereas an enchondroma does not (see Fig. 2-9*B*). An enchondroma often causes endosteal scalloping, whereas a bone infarct does not.

It is difficult, if not impossible, to differentiate an enchondroma from a chondrosarcoma. Clinical findings (primarily pain) serve as a better indicator than radiographic findings, and, indeed, pain in an apparent enchondroma should warrant surgical investigation. Periostitis should not be seen in an enchondroma either. Trying to differentiate an enchondroma from a chondrosarcoma histologically is also difficult, if not impossible at times. Therefore, biopsy of an apparent enchondroma should not be performed routinely for histologic differentiation. Magnetic resonance imaging (MRI) criteria for

FIGURE 2-7 **Adamantinoma.** A wild-looking mixed lytic and sclerotic lesion in the tibia that resembles fibrous dysplasia is classic for an adamantinoma. This lesion occurs only in the tibia and in the jaw and has some malignant potential. An adamantinoma should always be considered when a lesion resembling fibrous dysplasia is seen in the tibia.

FIGURE 2-8 **Enchondroma.** A benign lytic lesion in the hand is an enchondroma until proven otherwise. This is a common presentation of an enchondroma. Enchondromas in any other part of the body should contain some calcified chondroid matrix before they are included in the differential. However, calcified chondroid matrix is unusual in the phalanges.

Discriminators:

1. Must have calcification (except in phalanges)
2. No periostitis

Eosinophilic Granuloma

Eosinophilic granuloma (EG) is a form of histiocytosis X, the other forms being Letterer-Siwe disease and Hand-Schüller-Christian disease. Although these forms may be merely different phases of the same disease, most investigators categorize them separately. The bony manifestations of all three disorders are similar and are discussed in this book simply as eosinophilic granuloma, or EG.

EG, unfortunately for radiologists, has many appearances. It can be lytic or blastic, be well defined or ill defined (Figs. 2-11 and 2-12), have or not have a sclerotic border, and may or may not elicit a periosteal response.[2] The periostitis, when present, is typically benign in appearance (thick, uniform, wavy) but can be lamellated or amor-

benign versus malignant lesion includes lack of a soft tissue mass and no surrounding T2 high-signal edema in benign enchondromas.

Multiple enchondromas occur on occasion, and this condition has been termed Ollier's disease (Fig. 2-10A). It is not hereditary and does not have an increased rate of malignant degeneration. Older books say that Ollier's disease has a high rate of malignant degeneration; this is because any chondroid lesion can look "malignant" when a biopsy of it has been taken and needs to be correlated radiographically and clinically. The presence of multiple enchondromas associated with soft tissue hemangiomas is known as Maffucci's syndrome (see Fig. 2-10B). This syndrome also is not hereditary; however, it is characterized by an increased incidence of malignant degeneration of the enchondromas.

A

B

FIGURE 2-9 *A,* **Enchondroma.** A lesion in the distal femur is seen with irregular speckled calcification typical of chondroid matrix. This is virtually pathognomonic of an enchondroma. A chondrosarcoma could have an identical appearance but requires clinical symptomatology for consideration in the differential diagnosis. A bone infarct can be similar in appearance to an enchondroma. *B,* **Bone infarcts.** Bilateral lytic lesions in the femurs are noted with a densely calcified serpiginous border characteristic of bone infarcts. Compare these lesions with *A,* which does not have a well-defined serpiginous border. Often, the differentiation between bone infarcts as in this example and an enchondroma *(A)* is not so clearcut. (Case courtesy of Dr. Hideyo Minagi.)

phous. EG can mimic Ewing's sarcoma and appear as a permeative (multiple small holes) lesion.

How, then, can one distinguish EG from any of the other lytic lesions in this differential? Let me say outright that it is difficult to exclude EG from almost any differential of a bony lesion. Although some authorities say that up to 20% of EG cases occur in patients older than 30 years, others claim that it is rare in older age groups. I have seen only 1 or 2 cases of EG in patients older than 30 years and have seen at least 100 cases in children and young adults. Therefore, I find the 30 year cutoff point quite useful and am willing to exclude the diagnosis of EG in anyone older than 30 years. (I accept that I will miss the diagnosis in older age groups, but I hate to clutter up *every* differential with EG.)

EG is most often monostotic, but it can be polyostotic, and thus has to be included whenever multiple lesions are present. EG may or may not have a soft tissue mass associated with it, therefore the presence or absence of a soft tissue mass will not help in the differential diagnosis. In fact, I know of no entity in which the presence or absence of an associated soft tissue mass warrants inclusion or exclusion of a process from a differential. It is important to note the presence of a soft tissue mass (or its absence), but it will do little to narrow your differential diagnosis.

EG occasionally has a bony sequestrum (Fig. 2-13). Only three other entities have been described that, on occasion, have bone sequestra: osteomyelitis, lymphoma, and fibrosarcoma. Therefore, when a sequestrum is identified, these four entities should be considered (Table 2-2). (Another entity, osteoid osteoma, can sometimes have an appearance that mimics a sequestrum. See Chapter 8 for a more detailed discussion.) Clinically, EG may or may not be associated with pain; therefore, clinical history is noncontributory for the most part.

Discriminator: Patients must be younger than 30 years.

GIANT CELL TUMOR

A GCT is a somewhat controversial lesion with several schools of thought as to its radiographic appearance. I subscribe to the most widely used approach and will only briefly mention the other viewpoints.

First, it is important to realize that one is unable to tell, regardless of its radiographic appearance, if a GCT is benign or malignant. In fact, histologically, a GCT cannot be divided into either a benign or a malignant category. Most surgeons curettage and pack the lesions and consider them benign unless they recur. Even then they can still be benign and recur a second or third time. About 15% of GCTs are said to be malignant, on the basis

FIGURE 2-10 *A,* **Ollier's disease.** Multiple lytic lesions in the hand are seen in this patient, which are multiple enchondromas. This is known as Ollier's disease. *B,* **Maffucci's syndrome.** Multiple enchondromas associated with soft tissue hemangiomas are seen in the hand in this patient. This is Maffucci's syndrome. Note the multiple rounded calcifications in the soft tissues, which are phleboliths in the hemangiomas.

of their recurrence rate. Only rarely will GCTs metastasize. They metastasize to the lungs, and then should be characterized as malignant.

I use four radiographic criteria for diagnosing GCTs (Figs. 2-14 and 2-15). If any of these criteria are not met when looking at a lesion, I discard GCT from my differential diagnosis.

First, GCT occurs only in patients with closed epiphyses; this is valid in at least 98 to 99% of cases and is extremely useful. I will not diagnose GCT in a patient with open epiphyses.

Second, the lesion must be epiphyseal and abut the articular surface. There is disagreement over whether GCTs begin in the epiphysis or metaphysis, or in the physeal plate itself; however, except for rare cases, when radiologists see the lesions, they are epiphyseal and are flush against the articular surface. The metaphysis also has some of the tumor in it because the lesions are generally very large. I am not terribly interested in the embryogenesis of a lesion when I am looking at it as an unknown and a handful of surgeons are breathing down my neck wanting a differential diagnosis. I (and they) want to be able to intelligently say what it is or is not. Therefore, I don't get caught up in

the argument of where the lesion began. When you see a GCT, it will be epiphyseal. Perhaps more important, it should be flush against the articular surface of the joint. This occurs in 98 to 99% of GCTs[3]; therefore, if I have a lesion that is separated from the articular surface by a definite margin of bone, I will not include GCT in the diagnosis.

Third, these lesions are said to be eccentrically located in the bone, as opposed to being centrally placed in the medullary cavity. I don't find this to be a terribly helpful description, but it is one of the classic "rules" of a GCT. It is accurate; however, occasionally, the lesion is so large that it is difficult to tell whether it is really eccentric.

Fourth, the lesion must have a sharply defined zone of transition (border) that is not sclerotic. This is a helpful finding in GCT. The only places this does not apply are in flat bones, such as the pelvis, and the calcaneus.

Using these four "rules" will allow you to eliminate GCT from a list of differential possibilities with accuracy and assurance, when otherwise it would have to be included. Unwarranted inclusion of a lesion in a differential tends to clutter up the list and make it unnecessarily long.

FIGURE 2-11 **Eosinophilic granuloma.** A well-defined lytic lesion in the midshaft of a femur in a child. At biopsy this was shown to be eosinophilic granuloma. This is an entirely nonspecific pattern that could easily represent a focus of infection or one of several other processes. Because the lesion is present in a child, eosinophilic granuloma must be included in the differential diagnosis.

FIGURE 2-12 **Eosinophilic granuloma.** A predominantly lytic process with some sclerosis is seen in the proximal femur in a child. Again, this case would have a long differential diagnosis. Eosinophilic granuloma must be mentioned because the patient is younger than 30 years. In this example, the zone of transition is narrow and the lesion appears benign, but eosinophilic granuloma can have an aggressive appearance and mimic a sarcoma.

It is important to realize that the four criteria for a GCT apply only to GCTs and to no other lesion. For instance, I know of no other lesion that is dependent on whether the epiphyses are open or closed. No other lesion in any of my lists can be defined by whether the zone of transition is sclerotic (many lesions, such as nonossifying fibromas [NOFs], will usually have a sclerotic margin, but it doesn't occur often enough to include as a differential point). No other lesion must always abut the articular surface, and no other lesion has the classic description of being eccentrically placed (although several lesions, including NOF and chondromyxoid fibroma, are in fact eccentric in greater than 98% of cases).

Therefore, although these four criteria work nicely for GCT, they don't work at all for any other lesions. Residents have a tendency to apply these criteria to every lytic lesion encountered for the simple reason that they have learned the four criteria. Once one of the criteria is violated, the remainder don't even have to be used to eliminate a GCT. For instance, if a lytic lesion is found in the mid-diaphysis of a bone, GCT can be excluded. There is no need to check further to see if it is eccentric, if it has a nonsclerotic margin, or if the epiphyses are closed.

Again, these "rules" are greater than 95% effective and, in my experience, close to 99% effective, but only in long bones. Flat bones such as the pelvis and the calcaneus are exceptions. If one or two cases are found that don't fit the criteria, another pathologist should probably review the slides. Many pathologists refer to aneurysmal bone cysts (ABCs) as GCTs; hence, they have "GCTs" that don't obey *any* of the criteria. These pathologists may be correct, but they are not in the mainstream of what most people use for GCT criteria, either radiographically or histologically.

Discriminators (long bones only):

1. Epiphyses must be closed
2. Must abut the articular surface
3. Must be well defined with a nonsclerotic margin
4. Must be eccentric

FIGURE 2-13   **Eosinophilic granuloma.** A well-defined lytic lesion with a dense bony sequestrum in the proximal humerus of a child should conjure up the diagnosis of an infection. Eosinophilic granuloma also occasionally has a bony sequestrum (as in this example) and must be considered.

TABLE 2-2   **Entities That Can Present with a Sequestration**

Osteomyelitis
Eosinophilic granuloma
Malignant fibrous histiocytoma (includes
  fibrosarcoma and desmoids)
Lymphoma
Osteoid osteoma can mimic a sequestration

FIGURE 2-14   **Giant cell tumor.** A well-defined lytic lesion in the distal femur that has all four criteria typical for a giant cell tumor: (1) a well-defined but nonsclerotic zone of transition, (2) the epiphyses are closed, (3) the lesion is eccentrically placed in the bone, and (4) the lesion is epiphyseal and abuts the articular surface. If any one of these criteria were *not* adhered to, I would not include giant cell tumor in my differential.

NONOSSIFYING FIBROMA

NOF is probably the most common bone lesion encountered by radiologists. It reportedly occurs in up to 20% of children and spontaneously regresses so as to be seen only rarely after the age of 30. "Fibrous cortical defect" is a common synonym, although some people divide the two lesions on the basis of size, with fibrous cortical defect being shorter than 2 cm in length and NOF being longer than 2 cm. Histologically, these lesions are identical; therefore, it seems illogical to subdivide the lesion by its size.

NOFs are benign, asymptomatic lesions that typically occur in the metaphysis of a long bone emanating from the cortex (Figs. 2-16 to 2-18). They classically have a thin, sclerotic border that is scalloped and slightly expansile; however, this is a general description that probably applies to only 75% of the lesions. They do not have to have expansion or a scalloped or sclerotic border, and they are not limited to the metaphyses. Then how

will you recognize them? The best way is, again, to familiarize yourself with their general appearance by looking at examples in textbooks. That can be done in 15 minutes. It is important to recognize these lesions because they are what I call "don't touch" lesions—that is, the radiologist's diagnosis should be the final word, thereby supplanting a biopsy (see Chapter 4). These lesions are so characteristic that no logical differential diagnosis should be entertained, although a few entities can indeed occasionally simulate them.

I use age 30 as a cutoff point for NOFs. If the patient is older than 30 years, I will not include NOF in the differential diagnosis. The lesions must be asymptomatic and exhibit no periostitis, unless there is an antecedent history of trauma. NOFs routinely "heal" with sclerosis and eventually disappear (Figs. 2-19 and 2-20). During this "healing" period they can appear hot on a radionuclide bone scan because there is osteoblastic activity. Computed tomography (CT) scanning can show

FIGURE 2-15 **Giant cell tumor.** A typical example in the distal radius, which is a common location for giant cell tumor.

FIGURE 2-16 **Nonossifying fibroma.** A classic example of a nonossifying fibroma that is slightly expansile and lytic and has a scalloped, well-defined sclerotic border. The location in the metaphysis is characteristic. That the cortex is not well seen should not imply cortical destruction, but rather that the cortex has been replaced with benign fibrous tissue. This was an incidental finding in a patient who was asymptomatic.

apparent cortical breakthrough, which is really only fibrous tissue replacing cortex (Fig. 2-21). These lesions can occasionally get quite large (Fig. 2-22); therefore, growth or change in size will not alter the diagnosis. They are most commonly seen about the knee but can occur in any long bone.

The MRI appearance of an NOF is somewhat variable. Although they are essentially always low signal on T1-weighted imaging, they can have high or low signal on T2-weighted imaging (Fig. 2-23).

Discriminators:

1. Patient must be younger than 30 years
2. No periostitis or pain

OSTEOBLASTOMA

Osteoblastomas are rare lesions that could justifiably be excluded from this differential without the fear of missing a diagnosis more than once in your lifetime. Why, then, include them? The mnemonic FEGNOMASHIC would not have nearly the same ring without the extra vowel, so osteoblastoma remains.

Osteoblastomas have two appearances. They can look like large osteoid osteomas and are often called giant osteoid osteomas. Because osteoid osteomas are sclerotic lesions and do not resemble bubbly lytic lesions, this is not the type of osteoblastoma we are concerned with in this dif-

ferential. The other appearance simulates ABCs. These osteoblastomas are expansile, often having a soap bubble appearance (Fig. 2-24). If an ABC is being considered, an osteoblastoma should be as well. They most commonly occur in the posterior elements of the vertebral bodies, and about half of the cases demonstrate speckled calcifications. A classic radiology differential is that of an expansile lytic lesion of the posterior elements of the spine, and it includes osteoblastoma, ABC, and tuberculosis (Table 2-3).

TABLE 2-3 **Differential Diagnosis of Expansile Lytic Lesion in Posterior Elements of Spine**

Aneurysmal bone cyst
Osteoblastoma
Tuberculosis

FIGURE 2-17 **Nonossifying fibroma.** A well-defined expansile lytic lesion in the distal fibula is noted, which is characteristic for a nonossifying fibroma. The patient was asymptomatic, and the lesion was an incidental finding. The faint sclerosis seen in the lesion is secondary to the partial calcification or ossification of the matrix, which in a few years time will be complete as the lesion disappears.

Discriminator: Mentioned when ABC is mentioned.

METASTATIC DISEASE AND MYELOMA

Metastatic disease (mets) should be considered for any lytic lesion—benign or aggressive in appearance—in a patient older than 40 years. Mets can appear perfectly benign radiographically (Fig. 2-25), therefore it is not valid to say, "Since this lesion looks benign, it should not be a met." Most mets have an aggressive appearance and won't be in the FEGNO-MASHIC differential, but a significant number appear benign.

For statistical purposes I will not mention mets in a patient younger than 40 years. I will be correct more than 99% of the time using 40 years as a cut-off age. Otherwise, mets would have to be mentioned in every single case of a lytic lesion, and I'm trying to find ways to limit the list of differential

FIGURE 2-18 **Nonossifying fibroma.** A multilocular, expansile, well-defined lytic lesion in a long bone of a child who is asymptomatic. There is no need to do a biopsy for diagnosis because this is an obviously benign lesion and characteristic of a nonossifying fibroma.

possibilities. I'm not saying that mets does not occur in patients younger than 40 years, only that I'm willing to miss it (unless I'm given a history of a known primary neoplasm).

Myeloma can present as either solitary or multiple lytic lesions, which are more correctly called plasmacytomas (Fig. 2-26). I try to mention plasmacytoma separately from mets because it can occur in a slightly younger population (35 years is my cutoff) and can precede clinical or hematologic evidence of myeloma by 3 to 5 years. In general, there is no harm in lumping all mets, including myeloma, into one group and using older than 40 years as the limiting factor.

Virtually any metastatic process can present as a lytic, benign-appearing lesion; therefore, it serves no purpose to try to guess the source of the mets from its appearance. In general, lytic expansile mets tend to come from thyroid and renal tumors (Fig. 2-27). The only metastatic lesion that is said to always be lytic is renal cell carcinoma.

Discriminator: Patients must be older than 40 years.

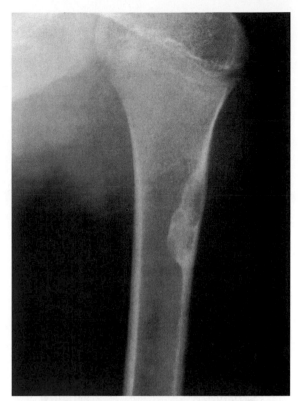

FIGURE 2-20 **Healing nonossifying fibroma.** A typical nonossifying fibroma in the proximal humerus of a child that is beginning to ossify. In a few years time this lesion will be essentially nonexistent.

FIGURE 2-19 **Healing nonossifying fibroma.** A lesion in a young adult characteristic of a nonossifying fibroma that is beginning to disappear or "heal." As these lesions are typically not seen in patients older than 30 years, it is thought that they ossify and then blend into the normal bone.

ANEURYSMAL BONE CYST

ABCs are the only lesions I know of that are named for their radiographic appearance. They are virtually always aneurysmal or expansile (Figs. 2-28 and 2-29). Rarely, an ABC will present before it is expansile, but this is unusual enough to not worry about. ABCs primarily occur in patients who are younger than 30 years, although occasionally one will be encountered in older patients. I use expansion and age younger than 30 years as fairly rigid guidelines, and seldom miss the diagnosis of ABC.

ABCs have a characteristic appearance on MRI examination with multiple fluid–fluid levels (Fig. 2-30). Although other entities can have fluid–fluid levels and ABCs don't always have them, the appearance is nevertheless so characteristic for an ABC that it is almost pathognomonic.

ABCs are, like GCTs, somewhat controversial. There are apparently two types of ABCs: a primary type and a secondary type. The secondary type occurs in conjunction with another lesion or from trauma, whereas a primary ABC has no known cause or association with other lesions. Secondary ABCs have been known to occur with GCTs, osteosarcomas, and almost any other lesion you can name; however, in my experience, this does not happen very often. As to occurring after trauma, I don't understand why they would be age-limited if trauma were the cause. Also, malignant tumors were once thought to occur after trauma because of the frequent antecedent history of trauma with malignant bone tumors. This is not currently seriously considered and is thought to be coincidental. I suspect that the relationship between ABCs and trauma is also coincidental, but this is mere speculation. This history of prior trauma should not make you think more or less of the proper diagnosis; therefore, it makes no difference when addressing an unknown lesion. Even in cases of myositis ossificans (a lesion known to be caused by trauma), a history of antecedent trauma is elicited only half of the time.

Patients typically present with ABCs because of pain. They occasionally can occur in the epiphyses, but there is no location in which they should

A

B

FIGURE 2-21 **Computed tomography (CT) of nonossifying fibroma.** An anteroposterior plain film *(A)* shows an expansile lytic lesion that was seen when this child had radiographs obtained for a sprained ankle. This is typical for a nonossifying fibroma. A CT scan was obtained through this lesion (for no good reason) *(B)*; it shows some disruption of the cortex *(arrow)*, which was felt to represent "cortical destruction." A biopsy of the lesion was therefore taken, and the lesion was found to be a nonossifying fibroma. This cortex is not destroyed but rather replaced with benign fibrous tissue.

FIGURE 2-22 **Large nonossifying fibroma.** This large, expansile, well-defined lytic lesion was noted in an asymptomatic 16-year-old patient, and a biopsy of the lesion was taken because it had grown over follow-up of several years. It was found to be a nonossifying fibroma. There is little justification for biopsy of this lesion, even though it is larger than most nonossifying fibromas.

be given more weight in the differential. As with osteoblastoma, they often occur in the posterior elements of the spine.

Discriminators:

1. Must be expansile
2. Patient must be younger than 30 years

SOLITARY BONE CYST

Solitary bone cysts are also called simple bone cysts or unicameral (one compartment) bone cysts. They are not necessarily unicameral, however. This is the only lesion in FEGNOMASHIC that is always central in location (Fig. 2-31). Many of the other lesions may be central, but a solitary bone cyst can be excluded if it is not. It is one of the few lesions that doesn't occur most commonly around the knees. Two thirds to three fourths of these lesions occur in the proximal humerus and proximal femur. By itself this fact isn't very helpful, because one third to one fourth of the lesions would be missed if only these areas were included.

FIGURE 2-23   MRI of nonossifying fibroma. An anteroposterior plain film (*A*) of a knee in a 16-year-old girl shows a benign appearing lytic lesion (*arrows*), which is consistent with an NOF. Sagittal T1- (*B*) and T2-weighted (*C*) images show a cortically based low signal lesion on both the T1 and the T2 sequences. This is characteristic for an NOF.

FIGURE 2-24 **Osteoblastoma.** A well-defined, expansile, lytic lesion in a 35-year-old patient that looks like an aneurysmal bone cyst. This is only one appearance of this rare lesion (the other appearance being a sclerotic lesion similar to an osteoid osteoma, although considerably larger).

Solitary bone cysts are usually asymptomatic unless fractured—a common occurrence (Fig. 2-32). Even when pathologic fractures occur, they rarely form periostitis. They usually occur in young patients, and it is unusual to see one in a patient older than 30 years. Although long bones are most commonly involved, solitary bone cysts have been described in almost every bone in the body. They begin at the physeal plate in long bones and grow into the shaft of the bone; therefore, they are not epiphyseal lesions. They can extend up into an epiphysis after the plate closes, but this is unusual. A fairly common location is in the calcaneus, where they have a characteristic triangular appearance (Fig. 2-33).

Discriminators:

1. Must be central
2. Patients must be younger than 30 years

HYPERPARATHYROIDISM (BROWN TUMORS)

Brown tumors of hyperparathyroidism (HPT) can have almost any appearance, from a purely

FIGURE 2-25 **Metastatic disease.** A typical renal metastasis is seen as a benign lytic lesion in the proximal femur in this patient.

lytic lesion to a sclerotic process (Fig. 2-34). Generally, when the patient's HPT is treated, the brown tumor undergoes sclerosis and will eventually disappear. If a brown tumor is going to be considered in the differential, additional radiographic findings of HPT should be seen. Subperiosteal bone resorption is pathognomonic for HPT and should be searched for in the phalanges (particularly the radial aspect of the middle phalanges), distal clavicles (resorption), medial aspect of the proximal tibias, and sacroiliac joints

FIGURE 2-26 **Plasmacytoma.** A large lytic lesion with a well-defined sclerotic border is seen in the left ilium in a patient with multiple myeloma. The ilium and sacrum are common sites for plasmacytomas.

FIGURE 2-27 **Metastatic renal cell carcinoma.** A bubbly expansile lesion of the proximal radius is noted that is typical for renal cell carcinoma metastasis. It is similar in appearance to an aneurysmal bone cyst.

(it has the appearance of bilateral sacroiliac [SI] joint erosive disease). Osteoporosis or osteosclerosis might suggest that renal osteodystrophy with secondary HPT is present, but subperiosteal resorption must be present; otherwise, brown tumor can be excluded from the differential.

Most authorities believe that brown tumors occur most commonly in primary HPT; however, because we see so many more patients with secondary HPT, more brown tumors are seen in patients with secondary rather than primary HPT.

Discriminator: There must be other evidence of HPT.

INFECTION

Unfortunately, there is no reliable way to radiographically exclude a focus of osteomyelitis (Figs. 2-35 and 2-36). It has a protean radiographic appearance and can occur at any location and in a patient of any age. It may or may not be expansile, have a sclerotic or nonsclerotic border, or have periostitis associated with it. Soft tissue findings such as obliteration of adjacent fat planes are noto-

FIGURE 2-28 **Aneurysmal bone cyst.** An expansile lesion in the diaphysis of the ulna in a young child that is typical for an aneurysmal bone cyst.

riously unreliable and even misleading, as tumors and EG can do the same thing.

When osteomyelitis occurs near a joint, if the articular surface is abutted, invariably the adjacent joint will be involved and show either cartilage loss or an effusion, or both (Fig. 2-37). This finding is not particularly helpful, because any lesion can cause an effusion, but it's the best example that I know.

When a sclerotic margin is present, infection usually causes it to be thick and ill defined or fuzzy on its outermost portion, but these findings are by no means always present and are only of limited usefulness.

If a bony sequestrum is present, osteomyelitis should be strongly considered. As previously mentioned, the only lesions described that demonstrate sequestra are infection, EG, lymphoma, and fibrosarcoma. Most cases of osteomyelitis, however, do not have sequestra, so this feature is also of limited use. Therefore, infection will be in almost every differential diagnosis of a lytic lesion,

FIGURE 2-29 **Aneurysmal bone cyst.** An expansile lytic lesion in a 25-year-old patient that is typical for an aneurysmal bone cyst. At first glance one might consider this typical for a giant cell tumor. However, note the sclerotic margins and that it does not abut the articular surface.

FIGURE 2-30 **Aneurysmal bone cyst (MRI).** An axial proton-density MR image through an expansile lytic lesion involving the posterior elements of a thoracic vertebral body reveals several fluid–fluid levels (*arrows*). This appearance is classic for an aneurysmal bone cyst.

FIGURE 2-31 **Solitary bone cyst.** A centrally placed lesion in the proximal femur that is classic for a solitary bone cyst.

which is all right, because it is one of the most common lesions encountered.

Discriminators: None.

CHONDROBLASTOMA

Chondroblastomas are among the easiest lesions to deal with because they occur only in the epiphyses (a handful of cases have been reported in the metaphyses—they are rare), and they occur almost exclusively in patients younger than 30 years (Fig. 2-38). What could be easier? Anywhere from 40 to 60% demonstrate calcification, therefore absence of calcification is not helpful. Presence of calcification is helpful so long as you can be sure that it's not detritus or sequestra from infection or EG (both of which can occur in the epiphyses). Because I can never be certain about the calcification, I don't worry about it.

The differential diagnosis of a lytic lesion in the epiphysis of a patient younger than 30 years is short and simple: (1) infection (most common), (2) chondroblastoma, and (3) GCT. (GCT has its own diagnostic criteria so it can usually be definitely ruled out or in.) This is an old, classic differential and probably takes care of 98% of epiphyseal lesions. If you want to be 99% certain,

FIGURE 2-33 Solitary bone cyst. A classic appearance of a solitary bone cyst in the calcaneus. This lesion in the calcaneus occurs only in this position (anterior to the midportion of the calcaneus and on the inferior border). Although other lesions could occur in this location, a solitary bone cyst of the calcaneus virtually never occurs away from this spot.

FIGURE 2-32 Solitary bone cyst. A pathologic fracture has occurred through this lesion in the proximal humerus. Its location and appearance are typical for a solitary bone cyst. Note the cortical fragments (*arrow*) produced from the fracture that have sunk to the bottom of this fluid-filled lesion. This is termed a "fallen fragment sign." No other lesion has been reported to have a fallen fragment sign; therefore, this is virtually pathognomonic.

you must add two more lesions—ABC (be certain it is expansile) and EG—and add mets and myeloma if the patient is older than 40 years. I no longer recommend using the longer differential because it just seems to cause confusion. Residents remember that there are three entities in the epiphyseal differential and then pick from the longer list of five entities, often leaving out the main things while including EG and ABC. Most of you have too much to commit to memory already without trying to stuff in a few rare presentations.

A caveat on epiphyseal lesions is to always consider the possibility of a subchondral cyst or geode, which has been described in four disease processes: (1) degenerative joint disease (the patient must have joint space narrowing, sclerosis, and osteophytes), (2) rheumatoid arthritis, (3) cal-

cium pyrophosphate dihydrate (CPPD) or pseudogout, and (4) avascular necrosis. Be certain no joint pathology that might indicate one of these processes is present, or an unnecessary biopsy of a geode might be performed on the basis of your differential of an epiphyseal lesion (see Chapter 4).

The carpal bones, the tarsal bones, and the patella have a tendency to behave like epiphyses as far as their differential diagnosis of lesions is concerned. Therefore, a lytic lesion in these areas has a similar differential as an epiphyseal lesion (Fig. 2-39).

Discriminators:

1. Patient must be younger than 30 years
2. Must be epiphyseal

CHONDROMYXOID FIBROMA

Like osteoblastoma, the chondromyxoid fibroma is such a rare lesion that failure to mention it is probably not going to result in missing more than one case in your lifetime. Why include it then? I recommend not including it, but it's part of the classic differential. If you do mention it, at least know what it looks like. Basically, chondromyxoid fibromas resemble NOFs (Fig. 2-40). Unlike NOFs, however, they can be seen in patients of any age. Patients can present with pain also, which does not occur with an NOF. Chondromyxoid fibromas have been reported to progress from a benign process to an aggressive and even malignant lesion, but this is extremely rare.

FIGURE 2-34 Brown tumor. An expansile lytic lesion in the fifth metacarpal that would have an extremely long differential diagnosis. Barely discernible is subperiosteal bone resorption on the radial aspect of the middle phalanges *(arrows)*. A second, smaller lytic lesion is seen at the proximal portion of the fourth proximal phalanx. It has a different appearance than the other lytic lesion, emphasizing how brown tumors can have almost any appearance. The multiplicity is typical for a brown tumor and limits the differential diagnosis. However, the finding of subperiosteal bone resorption makes any other diagnosis unlikely.

Discriminator: Mention when an NOF is mentioned.

ADDITIONAL POINTS

This chapter, in essence, has presented my differential for a benign lytic lesion of bone. It is probably 98% accurate, which is good enough for me. To increase the accuracy to 99%, it would be necessary to add a host of rare lesions, and the whole process would become too confusing for most residents to learn. If you have a favorite lesion that is not in this list, by all means add it. Likewise, if the list is already too cumbersome, forget about osteoblastoma and chondromyxoid fibroma. I'm unable to make it much simpler than that and still be reasonably accurate.

Some of the lesions I have omitted are intraosseous ganglion, pseudotumor of hemophilia, hemangioendothelioma, ossifying fibroma,

FIGURE 2-35 Brodie's abscess. A focus of infection that was chronic in this patient is seen in the distal tibia. The differential diagnosis for this lesion would be quite long if the subtle periostitis *(arrow)* and the clinical history of pain were not noted. Although this is a typical appearance for a chronic osteomyelitis (Brodie's abscess), infection can resemble almost anything.

FIGURE 2-36 Fungal infection. A lytic lesion with faintly seen sclerotic margins is noted in the distal femoral metaphysis and was found on biopsy to be blastomycosis.

FIGURE 2-37   Osteomyelitis with pyoarthritis. A plain film of the shoulder *(A)* in this child with shoulder pain shows a well-defined lytic lesion. Coronal T2-weighted MRI *(B)* shows high signal throughout the lesion, which extends through the cortex *(arrow)* into the joint. This is a typical appearance for osteomyelitis with extension into the joint.

intraosseous lipoma, glomus tumor, neurofibroma, plasma cell granuloma, and schwannoma. Others could be added to this list, of course, but they are best left to the pathologist—not the radiologist—for the diagnosis.

There are several features that are somewhat useful in separating out the various lesions in FEGNO-

MASHIC (see Table 2-1). For instance, if the patient is younger than 30 years, be sure to consider EG, chondroblastoma, NOF, ABC, and solitary bone cyst. This is not a differential diagnosis to list when faced with a lytic lesion in a patient younger than 30 years; several other lesions should be included in that differential. However, don't mention those five lesions

FIGURE 2-38   Chondroblastoma. A lytic lesion with a well-defined sclerotic margin in the proximal humeral epiphysis extending slightly across the epiphyseal plate. This is a typical appearance of a chondroblastoma. Almost half of all chondroblastomas have a small portion of the lesion extending across the physeal plate.

FIGURE 2-39   Chondroblastoma. A lytic lesion in the calcaneus that abuts the superior portion of the calcaneus has a fairly short differential diagnosis. The differential is essentially the same as in an epiphysis. On biopsy this lesion was found to be a chondroblastoma.

FIGURE 2-40   Chondromyxoid fibroma. This lytic lesion in the distal tibia with a well-defined sclerotic margin should have been a nonossifying fibroma. The differential diagnosis for this lesion would include several other entities, all of which are benign. Although a biopsy of this lesion probably should not have been done in this asymptomatic patient, it was performed, and the lesion was found to be a chondromyxoid fibroma.

in a patient older than 30 years; in this instance, those five lesions can probably be excluded.

If periostitis or pain is present (assuming no trauma, which can be a foolhardy assumption), you can exclude fibrous dysplasia, solitary bone cyst, NOF, and enchondroma. If the lesion is epiphyseal, the classic differential is infection, GCT, and chondroblastoma. ABC and EG also could be added to that differential but are not mandatory. If the patient is older than 40 years, add mets and myeloma and remove ABC, chondroblastoma, and EG from the epiphyseal list. Don't forget to consider a subchondral cyst or geode in epiphyseal lesions.

The epiphyseal differential tends to work also for the tarsal bones (especially the calcaneus), the carpal bones, and the patella. In the calcaneus, a unicameral bone cyst should also be considered and has a characteristic appearance and location (see Fig. 2-33). Apophyses are "epiphyseal equivalents" and have the same differential as epiphyses. The difference between an epiphysis and an apophysis is that epiphyses contribute to the length of a bone, whereas apophyses serve as ligamentous attachments.

A few findings that just don't seem to narrow the differential diagnosis are presence or absence of a soft tissue mass, expansion of the bone (except that it must be present in an ABC), a sclerotic or nonsclerotic border (except that it must be nonsclerotic in GCT), presence or absence of bony struts or compartments in the lesion, and size of the lesion.

There are a few lesions that I call "automatics" (Table 2-4)—that is, they need to be included automatically in almost every case. In patients younger than 30 years, EG and infection must be included in every differential of a lytic bone lesion. In fact, they should be mentioned in any case, except for trauma or arthritis, because they can have virtually *any* appearance—lytic, sclerotic, mixed, benign, aggressive, and so on. Hence, they can mimic almost any bone lesion. Make sure you give a thoughtful pause after inspecting the film—as if you really considered the pros and cons of mentioning them. This is gamesmanship, but it adds to your credibility. In patients older than 40 years, mets and infection are "automatics." No consideration for the appearance or location of the lesion needs to be made when using the automatics—simply find a lesion.

TABLE 2-4   "Automatics"

Younger than 30 years:
Eosinophilic granuloma
Infection
Older than 40 years:
Metastatic disease
Infection

DIFFERENTIAL DIAGNOSIS OF A SCLEROTIC LESION

Many lytic lesions spontaneously regress and are not usually seen in patients older than 30 years. When these lesions regress, they often fill in with new bone and have a sclerotic or blastic appearance. Therefore, when a sclerotic focus is identified in a 20- to 40-year-old patient, especially if it is an asymptomatic, incidental finding, the following lesions should be considered: NOF (Fig. 2-41), EG,

A   **B**

FIGURE 2-41   *A,* **Healing nonossifying fibroma.** This faintly sclerotic lesion in the proximal tibia of a 30-year-old asymptomatic patient is characteristic for a healing or disappearing nonossifying fibroma. Prior films showed a typical lytic nonossifying fibroma. *B,* **Healing nonossifying fibroma.** This densely sclerotic lesion in the posterior proximal tibia in a young asymptomatic patient was thought to represent an osteoid osteoma or osteomyelitis. Even though the patient was asymptomatic, a biopsy was performed. It revealed a nonossifying fibroma that had ossified. In a patient older than 40 years, metastatic disease would need to be considered.

FIGURE 2-42 Giant bone island. A large sclerotic lesion is seen in the right iliac bone, which could easily be mistaken for a focus of metastatic disease in a patient older than 40 years. This is a giant bone island and has the typical pattern of irregular "feathered" margins with the trabecula blending into the normal bone. The axis of the lesion is in the long axis of the bone or in the direction of the primary weight-bearing trabecula.

A   **B**

FIGURE 2-43 Resolving nonossifying fibroma. An anteroposterior plain film of a knee *(A)* in a 28-year-old man shows a sclerotic lesion in the metaphysis of the tibia. Coronal T1- *(B)* and T2-weighted *(C)* images of the knee reveal a lesion that on T1-weighted imaging has mixed high and low signal, consistent with fatty tissue in some areas, which is mixed high and low signal on the T2-weighted imaging. This is typical for a resolving NOF.

C

FIGURE 2-43, cont'd

solitary bone cyst, ABC, and chondroblastoma. Several other lesions should be included that can also appear sclerotic: fibrous dysplasia, osteoid osteoma, infection, brown tumor (healing), and perhaps a giant bone island (Fig. 2-42). As these lesions continue to resolve, they often will be seen to have varying amounts of normal fatty marrow (Fig. 2-43). They should not be mistakenly called intraosseous lipomas just because they contain fat, although no harm would come from that misdiagnosis—they are still benign, and in most cases it would be an incidental finding.

In any patient older than 40 years, the primary possibility for a sclerotic lesion is mets (now that I've passed 40, I'm seriously considering moving the age to 50).

REFERENCES

1. Gold RH, Ross SE, Brown RF, et al: "The radiologic learning file. An introduction to diagnostic radiology." Radiology 1972;104(1):27-31.
2. David R, Oria R, Kumar R, et al: Radiologic features of eosinophilic granuloma of bone. Pictorial essay. AJR 1989;153:1021-1026.
3. Dahlin D: Giant cell tumor of bone: Highlights of 407 cases. AJR 1985;144:955-960.

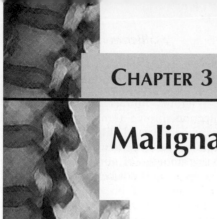

CHAPTER 3

Malignant Bone Tumors

Radiology residents have difficulty dealing with malignant bone tumors, and the difficulty gets worse in the years after residency. This is simply because malignant bone tumors, thankfully, are not common. Nevertheless, every radiologist will encounter one or two a year in most practices and should be able to recognize them and give a good differential diagnosis.

First, how do you recognize a malignant tumor and differentiate it from a benign process? This can be difficult and often it is impossible. Recognizing that it is *aggressive* is usually easy, but saying that it is *malignant* is another matter altogether. Processes such as infection and eosinophilic granuloma can mimic malignant tumors and are, of course, benign. They will often be included in the differential diagnosis of an aggressive lesion and with malignant tumors.

DIFFERENTIATION OF MALIGNANT FROM BENIGN

Which radiologic criteria are useful for determining malignant versus benign lesions? Standard textbooks and literature give four aspects of a lesion to be examined: (1) cortical destruction, (2) periostitis, (3) orientation or axis of the lesion, and (4) zone of transition.

Let me expound on each of these criteria and show why only the last one—the zone of transition—is up to 90% accurate.

Cortical Destruction

Often cortical bone is replaced by part of the noncalcified matrix (fibrous matrix or chondroid matrix) of benign fibro-osseous lesions and cartilaginous lesions. This can give the false impression of cortical destruction on plain films (Fig. 3-1) or computed tomography (CT). Also, benign processes such as infection and eosinophilic granuloma can cause extensive cortical destruction and mimic a malignant tumor. Aneurysmal bone cysts are known to cause such thinning of the cortex as to make it radiographically undetectable (Fig. 3-2). For these reasons I find cortical destruction to occasionally be misleading. Cortical destruction makes one think of a malignant lesion when using the Gestalt approach, but the lesion must also have other criteria for a malignant process, such as a wide zone of transition.

Periostitis

Periosteal reaction occurs in a nonspecific manner whenever the periosteum is irritated, whether it is irritated by a malignant tumor, a benign tumor, infection, or trauma. Callus formation in a fracture is actually just periosteal reaction of the most benign type. Periosteal reaction occurs in two types: benign (Fig. 3-3A and B) and aggressive (see Fig. 3-3C and D). The difference between the two is based more on the timing of the growth of the irritation than on whether the process causing the periostitis is malignant or benign. For example, a slow-growing benign tumor will cause thick, wavy, uniform, or dense periostitis because it is a low-grade chronic irritation that gives the periosteum time to lay down thick new bone and remodel into more normal cortex. A malignant tumor causes a periosteal reaction that is high-grade and more acute; hence, the periosteum does not have time to consolidate. It appears lamellated (onion skinned), amorphous, or even sunburst. If the irritation stops or diminishes, the aggressive periostitis will solidify and appear benign. Therefore, when periostitis is seen, the radiologist should try to characterize it into either a benign (thick, dense, wavy) type or an aggressive (lamellated, amorphous, sunburst) type.

Unfortunately, judging the lesion by its periostitis can be misleading. First, it takes considerable

FIGURE 3-1   **Apparent cortical destruction.** This benign chondroblastoma has noncalcified chondroid tissue replacing cortical bone in the proximal femur, which gives the lesion a destructive appearance. This is an example of cortical replacement rather than of cortical destruction, which can be confusing if one uses cortical destruction as an aggressive or malignant key in differential diagnosis. Note that the zone of transition is narrow, as one would expect in a benign lesion such as this.

experience to accurately characterize periostitis, because many times the reaction is not clearly benign or aggressive. Second, many benign lesions cause aggressive periostitis, such as infection, eosinophilic granuloma, aneurysmal bone cysts, osteoid osteomas, and even trauma. Seeing *benign* periostitis, however, can be helpful because malignant lesions will not cause benign periostitis. Some investigators with great experience in dealing with malignant bone tumors state that the only way benign periostitis can occur in a malignant lesion is if there is a concomitant fracture or infection. I have seen a few exceptions, but overall I think it is a valid statement.

Orientation or Axis of the Lesion

The orientation or axis of the lesion is a poor determinant of benign versus aggressive and seldom helps me to decide into which category the lesion should be placed. It has been said that if a lesion grows in the long axis of a long bone, rather than being circular, it is benign. Nonsense! Ewing's sarcoma, an extremely malignant lesion, usually has its axis along the shaft of a long bone. Conversely, many fibrous cortical defects are circular yet totally benign. I see no reason to even consider the axis of a lesion as part of its radiologic evaluation.

Zone of Transition

Without question, the zone of transition is the most reliable indicator in determining benign versus malignant lesions. Unfortunately, it also has some drawbacks.

The zone of transition is the border between the lesion and the normal bone. It is said to be narrow if it is so well defined that it can be drawn with a fine-point pen (Fig. 3-4). If it is imperceptible and cannot be clearly drawn, it is said to be wide (Fig. 3-5). Obviously, all shades of gray lie in between, but most lesions can be characterized as having either a narrow or a wide zone of transition. If the lesion has a sclerotic border, it, by definition, has a narrow zone of transition.

If a lesion has a narrow zone of transition, it is a benign process. The exceptions to that are rare, and I'm willing to miss them. If a lesion has a wide zone of transition, it is aggressive. Notice that I said aggressive and not malignant. As with aggressive periostitis, many benign lesions can have a wide zone of transition. A few of the same processes that can cause aggressive periostitis, and thereby mimic a malignant tumor, can have a wide zone of transition (i.e., infection and eosinophilic granuloma). They are aggressive in their radiographic appearance because they are fast-acting lesions. The zone of transition is usually easier to characterize than the periostitis, and it is always there to evaluate (or you wouldn't see a lesion), whereas many lesions, benign and malignant, have no periostitis. For these reasons the zone of transition is the most useful indicator of whether a lesion is benign or malignant.

A lesion that consists of multiple small holes is said to be permeative. It has no perceptible border, and therefore has a wide zone of transition. Round cell tumors such as multiple myeloma, reticulum cell sarcoma (primary lymphoma of bone), and Ewing's sarcoma are typical of this type of lesion. However, infection and eosinophilic granuloma (Fig. 3-6) can have the same appearance.

The zone of transition only applies to lytic or predominantly lytic lesions. A blastic or sclerotic lesion will always appear to have a narrow zone of transition and may erroneously get into the benign differential even if it is malignant.

It is critical to be aware that the zone of transition is a plain film-finding and cannot be used with magnetic resonance imaging (MRI). Most malignant tumors will appear to have narrow zones of transition on MRI examinations, which can mislead you into thinking a benign lesion is present (Fig. 3-7). The zone of transition can only be used with lytic lesions and on plain films.

FIGURE 3-2   *A,* **Aneurysmal bone cyst.** This benign lesion has thinned the cortex to such a degree as to make it imperceptible on a plain radiograph. As in Figure 3-1, this can be misconstrued as cortical destruction, giving the false impression of a malignant or very aggressive lesion. *B,* **Giant cell tumor.** This lesion in the proximal femur has expanded and thinned the cortex to such a degree that it is imperceptible on the plain film. *C,* On a computed tomography scan through this region a very thin cortex that was greatly expanded was identified. This giant cell tumor originated from the greater trochanter, which is an epiphyseal equivalent. Note that it has a well-defined but nonsclerotic zone of transition, as all giant cell tumors in long bones do.

FIGURE 3-3 **Benign periostitis.** *A,* An osteoid osteoma in the midshaft of the tibia has caused thick, wavy, dense periostitis, which is classic for a benign type of periostitis. Malignant lesions are incapable of forming this type of periostitis and should not be considered in the differential. This type of periostitis is basically indistinguishable from callus formation in a fracture. *B,* Thick, wavy periostitis *(arrows)* along the ilium in a child with a permeative lesion in the pelvis is characteristic for infection or eosinophilic granuloma. Ewing's sarcoma was initially considered in the differential; however, the benign periostitis would make a malignant lesion unlikely. Biopsy showed this lesion to be eosinophilic granuloma. *C,* **Aggressive periostitis.** Amorphous, sunburst periostitis with a Codman's triangle *(arrows)* in a patient with a mixed lytic-sclerotic lesion of the humerus, which on biopsy was shown to be Ewing's sarcoma. Although this type of periostitis is characteristic for a malignant lesion, it also could be seen with benign processes such as eosinophilic granuloma or infection. *D,* Lamellated, or onion-skinned, periostitis is characteristic of an aggressive process, such as in this patient with Ewing's sarcoma of the femur. Again, this aggressive type of periostitis could conceivably occur in a benign process such as infection or eosinophilic granuloma.

FIGURE 3-4   **Narrow zone of transition.** The border of normal bone with a lesion is known as the zone of transition. When, as in this example of a nonossifying fibroma, the border can be drawn with a fine-point pen it is said to be a narrow zone of transition, which is characteristic of a benign lesion. A narrow zone of transition may or may not have a sclerotic border.

FIGURE 3-6   **Permeative pattern.** A permeative pattern is defined as multiple, small, irregular holes in bone and indicates an aggressive process. Ewing's sarcoma typically has a permeative pattern; however, infection and eosinophilic granuloma, as in this example, also can have a permeative pattern. This is a fine-detailed film of the same case shown in Figure 3-3*B*.

FIGURE 3-5   **Wide zone of transition.** A lytic permeative process is seen in the midshaft of the femur in this patient. On biopsy it was found to be a malignant fibrous histiocytoma. The zone of transition in this lesion is said to be wide, because it cannot be easily drawn with a fine-point pen. A permeative lesion such as this, by definition, has a wide zone of transition.

DIFFERENTIATING TYPES OF TUMORS

Once it has been decided that a particular lesion is probably malignant, the differential is fairly straightforward. First of all, the list of malignant tumors is relatively short; and second, most tumors follow somewhat strict age groupings. Jack Edeiken, a famed skeletal radiologist, evaluated 4000 malignant bone tumors and found that they could be correctly diagnosed in 80% of cases just by using the patient's age! He basically divides the tumors into the decades when they will affect a patient; for example, osteosarcoma and Ewing's sarcoma are the only childhood primary malignant tumors of bone, and after the age of 40, only metastatic disease (mets), myeloma, and chondrosarcoma are common (Table 3-1). Although there are certainly outliers that are uncommon, these age guidelines are extremely useful. It is inappropriate to mention Ewing's sarcoma in a 40-year-old or mets in a 15-year-old patient. Obviously, if a 15-year-old patient has a known primary tumor, then mets must be considered—in fact, *any* bone lesion, regardless of its appearance, could be mets and would be suspicious in a patient with a known primary tumor.

MRI should be routinely used in the workup of malignant tumors. MRI will show the full bony and soft tissue extent and can identify the position

A

B

FIGURE 3-7 **Zone of transition on magnetic resonance imaging (MRI).** *A,* A T2-weighted MRI image of the knee in this child with knee pain shows a well-defined lesion *(arrow)* with a low signal border suggesting a narrow zone of transition with a sclerotic border. Because the knee pain was described as probably related to the menisci, this lesion was believed to be an incidental, benign process, such as a nonossifying fibroma. However, the plain film *(B),* obtained later, shows a barely discernible lytic lesion with a wide zone of transition *(arrow).* This lesion was, in fact, painful, and the differential diagnosis, based solely on the plain film, would include osteosarcoma—the eventual histologic diagnosis. The zone of transition can only be used on plain films; it is invalid on MRI.

Age, yr	Tumor
1-30	Ewing's sarcoma
	Osteosarcoma
30-40	Fibrosarcoma and malignant fibrous histiocytoma
	Malignant giant cell tumor
	Reticulum cell sarcoma
	Parosteal sarcoma
>40	Mets
	Myeloma
	Chondrosarcoma

TABLE 3-1　　Malignant Tumors and Patient Age

of the larger adjacent vessels, making angiography unnecessary. Routine use of gadolinium-diethylenetriamine penta-acetic acid (Gd-DTPA) with tumors does not appear to be justified, because it currently seems to give no more information than noncontrast-enhanced studies do.

Rather than give a description of characteristics of every malignant tumor, which is available in any of the leading skeletal radiology textbooks, let me make a few points on many of the primary malignant tumors of bone that I think may be helpful in their diagnosis.

Osteosarcoma. The most common malignant primary bone tumor is an osteosarcoma. Although it typically occurs toward the end of a long bone, it may occur anywhere in the skeleton, and does so with enough frequency so that location is not a helpful discriminator. Osteosarcomas are usually destructive, with obvious sclerosis present from either tumor new bone or reactive sclerosis (Figs. 3-8 and 3-9); however, on occasion they can be entirely lytic (Fig. 3-10). These are usually so-called telangiectatic osteosarcomas. There are many types and classifications of osteosarcomas, but it serves little purpose to the radiologist to try to distinguish among most of them.

These tumors occur almost exclusively in patients younger than 30 years. Although some textbooks claim there is a second peak of osteosarcomas in patients about 60 years old, I, and others, do not believe this to be correct. Some osteosarcomas occur in older patients who have malignant degeneration of Paget's disease, and some occur secondary to prior irradiation; but *de novo* osteosarcomas in the older age group are distinctly rare.

Parosteal Osteosarcoma. A type of osteosarcoma that should be distinguished from the central osteosarcoma is the parosteal osteosarcoma. The parosteal osteosarcoma originates from the periosteum of the bone and grows outside the bone (Fig. 3-11). It often wraps around the diaphysis without breaking through the cortex. It occurs in an older age group than the central osteosarcomas

FIGURE 3-8 Osteosarcoma. An extremely sclerotic lesion in the proximal tibia of a child is noted, which is characteristic for an osteogenic sarcoma.

and is not as aggressive. Treatment used to consist of merely shaving the tumor off the bone where it originated; however, recurrence rates were so high that currently wide-bloc excisions are performed. Once a parosteal osteosarcoma violates the cortex of the adjacent bone, some consider it to be as aggressive as a central osteosarcoma and is treated in a similar fashion (i.e., amputation or radical excision). Therefore, the radiologist needs to evaluate the lesion for invasion of the adjacent cortex to help determine treatment and prognosis. This is best done with CT scan or MRI (see Fig. 3-11*B* and *C*).

A common location for parosteal osteosarcomas to arise from is the posterior femur, near the knee. A lesion that can mimic an early parosteal osteosarcoma in this location is a so-called cortical desmoid (Fig. 3-12). A cortical desmoid is an avulsion injury that is totally benign but can appear somewhat aggressive. Unfortunately, it can appear malignant histologically, so biopsy can lead to disastrous consequences. Amputations for benign cortical desmoids which were mistaken for malignancies have occurred. (See Chapter 4 for further points on cortical desmoids.) Another lesion

that can be mistaken for a parosteal osteosarcoma is an area of myositis ossificans (Fig. 3-13). Like cortical desmoids, areas of myositis ossificans can be histologically mistaken for malignancies with disastrous consequences. Therefore, differentiation is vital. Fortunately, differentiation between parosteal osteosarcoma and myositis ossificans is fairly easily done radiographically. (See Chapter 4 for differential points between parosteal osteosarcoma and myositis ossificans.)

Another type of osteosarcoma that often gets mentioned by residents in their differentials of a parosteal osteosarcoma is a periosteal osteosarcoma. It should not get such attention. First, it's extremely rare, with fewer than 50 such lesions reported in the literature. Second, and most significantly, periosteal osteosarcomas do not resemble parosteal osteosarcomas (Fig. 3-14). Therefore, mentioning both of these lesions in the same differential is inappropriate and simply means that the resident doesn't know what a periosteal osteosarcoma looks like. It's such a rare lesion that I teach residents not to worry about it—don't mention it. Radiology is hard enough without remembering all the rare lesions that might be seen once in a lifetime, if at all.

Ewing's Sarcoma. The classic Ewing's sarcoma is a permeative (multiple small holes) lesion in the diaphysis of a long bone in a child (see Fig. 3-3*D*). However, only about 40% of these tumors occur in the diaphysis, with the remainder being metaphyseal, diametaphyseal, or in flat bones. They do tend to be found primarily in children and adolescents, although a significant number occur in patients who are in their 20s, especially in flat bones. Although most often permeative in appearance, they can elicit reactive new bone, which can give the lesion a partially sclerotic or "patchy" appearance (Figs. 3-3*C*, 3-15, and 3-16). Ewing's sarcomas often have an onion-skinned type of periostitis, but they can also have periostitis that is sunburst or amorphous in character (see Fig. 3-16). Rarely, if ever, will a Ewing's sarcoma have benign-appearing periostitis (thick, uniform, or wavy). If benign periostitis is present, other lesions should be considered instead, such as infection or eosinophilic granuloma.

A knee jerk differential diagnosis for a permeative lesion in a child should be Ewing's sarcoma, infection, and eosinophilic granuloma. These three entities can appear radiologically identical. I exclude Ewing's sarcoma from the differential if I can see definite benign periostitis, or if I can see a definite sequestrum of bone. In this differential list only eosinophilic granuloma and infection can have benign periostitis or a sequestrum. Presence or absence of a soft tissue mass is not helpful in distinguishing among these three lesions. Presence of

FIGURE 3-9 **Osteosarcoma.** *A,* A subtle sclerotic lesion is seen in the left ilium adjacent to the sacroiliac joint that was initially diagnosed as osteitis condensans ilii, a benign entity. Because of persistent pain, the patient returned for a follow-up visit, and a small amount of cortical destruction on the pelvic brim was noted *(arrow). B,* A computed tomography scan was performed, which showed a large soft tissue mass and tumor new bone around the ilium, which is characteristic for an osteogenic sarcoma.

symptoms is not helpful, because all three entities can be symptomatic; however, it would be unusual to find an asymptomatic Ewing's sarcoma.

Chondrosarcoma. Chondrosarcomas have a number of appearances that at times make them difficult to diagnose with any assurance. They most frequently occur in patients older than 40 years. An eminent bone radiologist once told me

that if a pathologist makes the diagnosis of chondrosarcoma in a child, get another pathologist. Although it is uncommon, chondrosarcomas occasionally do occur in children; usually they are from malignant degeneration of an osteochondroma (Fig. 3-17) but they do not have to be. I reserve the diagnosis of a chondrosarcoma for patients older than 40 years unless the patient has an obvious

FIGURE 3-10   **Lytic osteosarcoma.** An ill-defined lytic lesion was noted in the proximal tibia of a 20-year-old patient with pain. The lesion had a differential diagnosis of eosinophilic granuloma, infection, Ewing's sarcoma, and osteogenic sarcoma. Biopsy showed it to be a lytic osteogenic sarcoma.

enchondroma or osteochondroma that is painful or has a destructive appearance.

Probably the most difficult lesion for a pathologist to deal with is an enchondroma. It can be extremely difficult histologically to differentiate a low-grade chondrosarcoma from an enchondroma. Because low-grade chondrosarcomas do not metastasize, some pathologists call them "active enchondromas." The diagnosis of chondrosarcoma usually initiates radical excision and therapy, although it is debatable (and somewhat controversial) as to whether a low-grade chondrosarcoma is even a malignant tumor. For these reasons I usually reserve the diagnosis of "possible chondrosarcoma" for those lesions that are painful or show definite aggressive characteristics, such as periostitis and destruction. The truth of the matter is that neither radiologists nor pathologists can reliably distinguish between enchondromas and many chondrosarcomas (Fig. 3-18). MRI can be helpful in

distinguishing between a benign enchondroma and a chondrosarcoma. If a soft tissue mass or edema is present, it is unlikely to be an enchondroma.

Chondrosarcoma should be considered in the diagnosis anytime there is a lytic, destructive lesion with amorphous, snowflake calcification in an older patient (>40 years) (Fig. 3-19). Without the presence of the calcified chondroid matrix the lesion is indistinguishable from any other aggressive lytic lesion, such as mets, plasmacytoma, fibrosarcoma, malignant fibrous histiocytoma (MFH), or infection. Usually the radiologist can only give a long differential diagnosis such as the list just given, which is entirely acceptable. A biopsy of the lesion will have to be performed at any rate, so it is not necessary for the radiologist to make the diagnosis. This is the case with most malignant tumors. The radiologist does play an important role, however, in suggesting additional lesions that might masquerade as malignancies and in imaging the lesion to show such features as the full extent, the presence of a soft tissue component, and metastases. As mentioned earlier, MRI plays an invaluable role in this regard and should be performed on every potential malignant bone lesion.

Malignant Giant Cell Tumor.   Giant cell tumors (GCTs) are rarely malignant if mets is the marker for malignancy. It is said that approximately 15% of GCTs are malignant; however, this is based on how often they recur, which is not a valid marker for malignant. Unfortunately, there does not seem to be any way to foretell which GCT will become malignant. Benign and malignant GCTs appear radiologically identical (see Chapter 2). They also are histologically the same. So how is the diagnosis made? If metastases (usually to the lung) occur, or if a previously resected GCT recurs, the tumor is considered malignant. Malignant GCTs tend to occur primarily in the fourth decade of life.

Fibrosarcoma.   Fibrosarcomas are lytic malignant tumors that do not produce osteoid or chondroid matrix. They usually do not elicit reactive new bone and, therefore, are almost always lytic in appearance. This lytic appearance may take any form, from permeative to moth-eaten (Fig. 3-20) to a fairly well-defined area of lysis (Fig. 3-21). This can make radiographic diagnosis difficult.

The age range for fibrosarcomas is quite broad, but they tend to predominate in the fourth decade. Fibrosarcoma (and its cousins—MFHs and desmoids) and lymphoma are the only malignant tumors that can, on occasion, have a bony sequestrum. Also, fibrosarcomas, desmoids, and MFHs tend to be the only tumors that are not consistently high in signal on T2-weighted MR images (Fig. 3-22).

FIGURE 3-11   **Parosteal osteogenic sarcoma.** *A,* A lateral film of the distal femur shows a large calcific mass with an ill-defined, fluffy, calcific periphery growing off the posterior femur. The location and appearance are characteristic for a parosteal osteogenic sarcoma. *B,* A computed tomography scan through this lesion shows cortical and medullary involvement, which indicates a more sinister lesion, with treatment and prognosis similar to that of a central osteogenic sarcoma. Without intramedullary involvement, a parosteal sarcoma has a favorable prognosis. *C,* A proton density magnetic resonance image in another patient with a parosteal osteosarcoma shows how the vessels *(arrow)* can be easily identified in relation to the tumor. In this example, the vessels are displaced posteriorly by the tumor.

FIGURE 3-12 Cortical desmoid. Irregular periostitis (*arrows*) off the medial supracondylar ridge of the distal femur is pathognomonic for a small avulsion of the adductor muscles and is called a cortical desmoid. Biopsy of this lesion can easily result in a mistaken diagnosis of a sarcomatous lesion and should, therefore, be avoided. A cortical desmoid should not be confused with an early parosteal osteogenic sarcoma on radiographs, because this will then lead to an unnecessary biopsy, perhaps with dire consequences. An incidental finding is a nonossifying fibroma seen just proximal to the cortical desmoid.

FIGURE 3-13 Myositis ossificans. This lesion often is confused with parosteal osteogenic sarcoma, because at first glance it has a close resemblance. However, myositis ossificans, as in this example, will demonstrate calcification that is densest in the periphery and well defined, whereas parosteal osteogenic sarcoma has calcification that is most concentrated centrally and ill defined in the periphery. Myositis ossificans is another lesion that can be confused with a malignant lesion on biopsy and, therefore, should be radiographically rather than surgically diagnosed.

Malignant Fibrous Histiocytoma. Originally classified as fibrosarcoma by most pathologists, MFH has come into its own grouping in the last few decades. MFHs are much more common than fibrosarcomas. Whereas we see one or more MFHs every week, I have not encountered a fibrosarcoma in several years. Radiologically, an MFH appears identical to a fibrosarcoma—lytic lesions with variations extending from permeative (Fig. 3-23) to fairly well defined. Like fibrosarcomas, they may, on occasion, have a bony sequestrum. Anytime fibrosarcoma is mentioned, MFH should be included, because they can look identical radiographically.

Desmoid. A desmoid tumor (not to be confused with a cortical desmoid; see Chapter 4) is a half-grade fibrosarcoma. It has also been called a desmoplastic fibroma or aggressive fibromatosis. These lesions, like fibrosarcoma, are lytic but are usually fairly well defined because of their slow growth. They often have benign periostitis present that has thick spicules, or "spikes," and normally have a multilocular appearance with thick septa (Figs. 3-24 and 3-25). They are slow growing and seldom metastasize, but they can exhibit inexorable tumor extension into surrounding soft tissues with disastrous results. Like fibrosarcoma and MFHs, these lesions can exhibit a bony sequestrum (see Fig. 3-24).

Primary Lymphoma of Bone (Reticulum Cell Sarcoma). A rare neoplasm, primary lymphoma of bone (formerly called reticulum cell sarcoma) has a radiologic appearance identical to that of Ewing's sarcoma (i.e., a permeative or moth-eaten pattern) (Fig. 3-26). It tends to occur in an older age group than does Ewing's sarcoma, and whereas the patient who has Ewing's sarcoma is typically systemically symptomatic, the patient who has primary lymphoma of bone is often asymptomatic. In fact, primary lymphoma of bone is the only malignant tumor that can involve a large amount of bone while the patient is systemically asymptomatic.

FIGURE 3-14 **Periosteal osteogenic sarcoma.** Unlike the parosteal osteosarcoma, the periosteal osteogenic sarcoma does not have large amounts of calcification in soft tissues. It typically has a saucerized configuration with periostitis that resembles hair on end or is sunburst, as in this example. Although this lesion is malignant, it inexplicably will not invade the medullary space. Although parosteal and periosteal sarcomas originate from the same point and have similar names, they do not have a similar radiographic appearance.

FIGURE 3-15 **Ewing's sarcoma.** A mixed lytic-sclerotic lesion in the femur of a child with periostitis that is amorphous and sunburst, such as in this example, is characteristic of a Ewing's sarcoma. An osteosarcoma could have a similar appearance.

Metastatic Disease. Metastatic lesions must be included in *any* differential diagnosis of a bone lesion in a patient older than 40 years. They can have virtually any appearance: they can mimic a benign lesion (see Chapter 2) or a primary bone tumor. Judging the origin of the tumor from the appearance of the metastatic focus can be difficult, if not impossible, although some appearances are fairly characteristic. For instance, multiple sclerotic foci in a male patient are probably prostatic metastases (Fig. 3-27), although lung, bowel, or almost any other organ tumor could present in the same way. In a female patient the same picture would probably result from breast metastases. The only primary tumor that virtually never presents with blastic mets is renal cell carcinoma. Typically, an expansile lytic metastasis should be either renal or thyroid in origin (Fig. 3-28).

Myeloma. Like metastases, myeloma should be considered only in a patient older than 40 years, although some radiologists use age 35 years for the lower limits of myeloma. Myeloma typically has a diffuse permeative appearance that can mimic a Ewing's sarcoma or a primary lymphoma of bone (Fig. 3-29). It frequently involves the calvarium (Fig. 3-30). Because of the age criteria, Ewing's sarcoma and myeloma are not in the same differential, however. Rarely, myeloma can present with multiple sclerotic foci that resemble diffuse mets. Myeloma is one of the only lesions that is not characteristically "hot" on a radionuclide bone scan; therefore, radiologic "bone surveys" are performed instead of radionuclide bone scans when evidence of myeloma is found clinically.

Myeloma has two different appearances in the spine on CT scans. Acute myeloma appears as one would imagine—it has a "Swiss cheese" pattern of

FIGURE 3-16 **Ewing's sarcoma.** This is a predominantly sclerotic process with large amounts of sunburst periostitis in the diaphysis of a femur that, on biopsy, was found to be Ewing's sarcoma.

FIGURE 3-17 **Chondrosarcoma.** A large soft tissue mass with typical chondroid matrix is seen in this young adult with a history of multiple osteochondromatosis. A sessile osteochondroma is seen off the proximal humerus, and another osteochondroma is seen protruding off the scapula *(arrow)*. The chondrosarcoma in the axilla presumably arose from a prior benign osteochondroma that has undergone malignant degeneration.

multiple holes (Fig. 3-31). Chronic or long-standing myeloma, however, has a wild-looking pattern of dense, thick bony struts that resembles Paget's disease (Fig. 3-32). This is a characteristic "Aunt Minnie" on CT but is not appreciated on plain films—both the acute and chronic myeloma simply appear osteopenic on plain films.

Occasionally, myeloma will present with a lytic bone lesion called a plasmacytoma. This lesion can mimic any lytic bone lesion, benign or aggressive, in its appearance; it can precede other evidence of myeloma by up to 3 years. It can be solitary or multiple, although some insist it must be solitary to be considered a plasmacytoma, and when it is multifocal it is myeloma. Whatever. It has an appearance on MRI in the vertebral body that is virtually pathognomonic. It resembles the cadaveric section of a brain with which every medical student is familiar, hence the description, "mini-brain" appearance (Fig. 3-33).

Soft Tissue Tumors. Most radiology residents feel uneasy when faced with the differential diagnosis of a soft tissue tumor. They will give elabo-

FIGURE 3-18 **Chondrosarcoma.** Typical snowflake, punctate, amorphous calcification in the proximal humerus is seen, which is typical of an enchondroma. The patient, however, had pain associated with this lesion, and on biopsy it was found to be a chondrosarcoma. (Courtesy Dr. Tomas Jimenez-Robinson.)

FIGURE 3-19 **Chondrosarcoma.** An amorphous, irregular calcification is seen in a lesion arising in the ischium (*arrow*). This is fairly typical for a chondrosarcoma.

FIGURE 3-20 **Fibrosarcoma.** An ill-defined lytic lesion that is permeative or moth-eaten is seen in the diaphysis of the femur. On biopsy it was shown to be a fibrosarcoma.

rate description with plenty of pertinent and not-so-pertinent negatives, such as "no calcifications are seen," "no bony destruction is noted," and "no obliteration of fat planes is apparent." Then, when faced with finally giving a differential, few can give an authoritative list of the possibilities. The reason for this is quite simple: there is no authoritative, useful differential for soft tissue tumors, whether there is calcification, bony destruction, fat plane involvement, or whatever. You can play the odds and mention the two most common soft tissue tumors, MFH and liposarcoma, as the best candidates, but any cell type can produce a benign or malignant tumor and mimic any other soft tissue tumor. A lipoma can be identified by the appearance of fat, but a liposarcoma may or may not have fat present. Therefore, we are left to give descriptions of size and extent, and let the pathologist tell us the rest. Most of us are uncomfortable with this approach because our training has been to derive an answer—or at least a listing of probable lesions. This is just not possible for soft tissue tumors.

Following are a few words about soft tissue tumors that may be helpful: as mentioned earlier, liposarcomas do not have to have fat visible in the tumor. There are at least three subtypes of liposarcomas, two of which have only small amounts of fat present. Synovial sarcomas, or synoviomas, only rarely, if ever, originate in a joint. They are often adjacent to joints. There are no malignant tumors that routinely need to be considered in the differential diagnosis of joint lesions. Synovial osteochondromatosis is a benign joint lesion that occurs from metaplasia of the synovium and leads to multiple calcific loose bodies in a joint. This can histologically mimic a chondrosarcoma; therefore, it is best diagnosed radiographically, because it has a pathognomonic radiographic appearance (Fig. 3-34). Up to 30% of the time, however, the loose bodies do not calcify, and the lesion then can mimic pigmented villonodular synovitis (PVNS) on plain films. With MRI synovial osteochondromatosis can have a "tumefactive" appearance, with all the loose bodies packed together so tightly that it resembles a solid mass in the joint (Fig. 3-35). I have seen two cases where MRI suggested a tumor, a subsequent biopsy was called chondrosarcoma, and amputation was then performed. This assures a great 5-year survival rate, but the diagnosis should be made before a biopsy is performed so that a tumor is not in the differential.

PVNS also is a benign synovial soft tissue process that causes joint swelling, pain, and, occasionally, joint erosions (Fig. 3-36). Calcifications are virtually never associated with it. Hemangiomas often have phleboliths associated with them and often cause "cortical holes" in adjacent bone that mimic

FIGURE 3-21 **Fibrosarcoma.** A large, fairly well-defined destructive process of the entire right iliac wing is noted. On biopsy this was shown to be a fibrosarcoma. Fibrosarcomas can be very slow growing and will occasionally have a narrow zone of transition, such as in this figure.

A   **B**

FIGURE 3-22 **Desmoid.** A large soft tissue mass (*arrows*) is seen in the right buttock, which is low signal on both the T1-(*A*) and T2-weighted (*B*) images. This is typical for a soft tissue desmoid tumor.

FIGURE 3-23 **Malignant fibrous histiocytoma.** A moth-eaten or permeative process in the distal femur, with some involvement of the posterior cortex, is seen on this lateral radiograph. In a patient younger than 30 years, a Ewing's sarcoma, eosinophilic granuloma, or infection would be the differential diagnosis. In a patient older than 40 years, infection and MFH would be more common. A reticulum cell sarcoma could have a similar appearance.

FIGURE 3-24 **Desmoid tumor.** A lytic destructive process involving both bones of the distal forearm is noted, with at least one portion demonstrating a sequestrum *(arrow)*. A desmoid tumor is a fibrosarcoma-like lesion, and fibrosarcomas are known to occasionally demonstrate bony sequestra in the same manner as will osteomyelitis, lymphoma, and eosinophilic granuloma.

A   **B**

FIGURE 3-25 **Desmoid tumor.** *A* and *B,* A multilocular, heavily septate, destructive lytic lesion of the distal femur is noted, which is fairly characteristic for a desmoid tumor. The thick septa and narrow zone of transition are characteristic of a benign process, whereas the Codman's triangle and the large amount of bony destruction indicate an aggressive process.

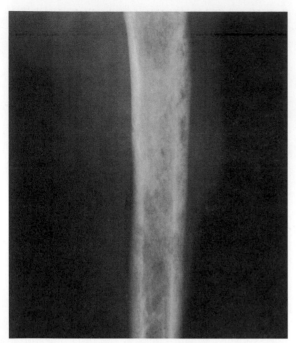

FIGURE 3-26 **Primary lymphoma of bone.** A diffuse permeative pattern throughout the humerus in this 35-year-old patient is characteristic of primary lymphoma of bone.

FIGURE 3-28 **Metastatic renal cell carcinoma.** A lytic lesion in the diaphysis of the femur is noted, which is characteristic for renal cell carcinoma. Up to one third of renal cell carcinomas initially present with a bony metastasis. Renal cell carcinoma virtually never presents with a blastic metastatic focus.

FIGURE 3-27 **Metastatic prostate carcinoma.** Diffuse blastic metastases are seen throughout the pelvis and proximal femurs, with a lytic destructive lesion seen in the right proximal femur. Prostate metastases tend to be blastic, but as shown here occasionally they can be lytic.

FIGURE 3-31 Computed tomography (CT) appearance of multiple myeloma. An axial CT image through a vertebral body in a patient with multiple myeloma shows a "Swiss cheese" appearance typical for this disease in the acute stages.

FIGURE 3-29 Multiple myeloma. A diffuse moth-eaten pattern is seen throughout the diaphysis of the femur in this 45-year-old patient, which is characteristic for myeloma. Primary lymphoma of bone could have a similar appearance.

FIGURE 3-30 Multiple myeloma. A lateral view of the skull shows multiple lytic lesions in the calvarium, which is a characteristic appearance of multiple myeloma.

FIGURE 3-32 Computed tomography (CT) appearance of chronic multiple myeloma. An axial CT image through a vertebral body in a patient with long-standing multiple myeloma shows the typical appearance of hypertrophied bony struts giving a wild-looking pattern somewhat resembling Paget's disease.

FIGURE 3-34 Synovial osteochondromatosis. Multiple calcific loose bodies in a hip joint such as this are virtually pathognomonic for synovial osteochondromatosis. Notice the erosions in the acetabulum. In up to 30% of cases the loose bodies are nonossified. When nonossified, this process is indistinguishable from pigmented villonodular synovitis on plain films.

A **B**

FIGURE 3-33 Magnetic resonance imaging appearance of plasmacytoma. Axial proton density (*A*) and T2-weighted (*B*) images through a vertebral body with a plasmacytoma show a characteristic, if not pathognomonic, appearance of a "mini-brain," which is seen only with plasmacytoma.

FIGURE 3-35 **Tumefactive synovial osteochondromatosis.** *A,* A plain film of the shoulder shows a partially calcified mass that is eroding the medial aspect of the humerus. Coronal proton density *(B)* and T2-weighted *(C)* images of the shoulder reveal a large mass encircling the humeral head, which was interpreted as a sarcoma. A biopsy was performed and called "chondrosarcoma," which resulted in a forequarter amputation. The intra-articular nature of the mass was not appreciated until after the radical surgery, when it was correctly recognized as synovial chondromatosis.

a permeative pattern (Fig. 3-37). The permeative pattern of round cell lesions occurs in the intramedullary or endosteal part of the bone and can be differentiated from "cortical holes" by the intact cortex (see Chapter 7). Atypical synovial cysts, such as Baker's cysts around the knee, can present as a soft tissue mass and result in an unnecessary biopsy. On CT scans these lesions may not be appreciated as fluid-filled lesions, and their association with a joint can be easily overlooked. MRI will demonstrate a

very high-signal intensity with T2 weighting and may show some fluid in the adjacent joint with an identical signal (Fig. 3-38). Differentiation of a solid mass from a ganglion is one of the few uses of Gd-DTPA in musculoskeletal MRI. A solid tumor will diffusely enhance with gadolinium, whereas a ganglion will have rim enhancement only. Intravenous contrast should be given whenever a mass that looks like a fluid collection or cyst is seen in a location atypical for a cyst or ganglion. Two

FIGURE 3-36 **Pigmented villonodular synovitis (PVNS).** Large erosions in the femoral head and acetabulum are characteristic for PVNS; however, nonossified synovial osteochondromatosis could present like this.

FIGURE 3-37 **Hemangioma.** Multiple, irregular lytic lesions, predominantly cortical in nature, are seen in the tibia in this patient with a soft tissue mass. Cortical holes such as this occur almost exclusively in radiation and soft tissue hemangioma. Note the phleboliths in the posterior soft tissues *(arrows)*, which often are seen in hemangioma and make this an easy diagnosis.

A

FIGURE 3-38 **Atypical synovial cyst.** *A,* Computed tomography scan through the distal femurs in a patient with a soft tissue mass around the right knee shows a multilocular soft tissue mass adjacent to the distal right femur *(arrows).*

B   **C**

F<small>IGURE</small> **3-38, cont'd**   *B,* A magnetic resonance imagine (MRI) examination with T1 weighting through the same area as imaged in *A* shows intermediate-intensity signal in a multilocular soft tissue mass. *C,* An MRI examination with T2 weighting shows high-intensity signal in the lesion, which is characteristic for fluid. This was an atypical synovial cyst arising from the knee joint.

tumors that typically mimic fluid on T2-weighted MR images are synovial sarcoma and neural tumors (neurofibromas and schwannomas) (Fig. 3-39).

A common mistake many make in giving IV contrast with MRI examination of tumors is to fat-suppress the postcontrast images and compare them with the non-fat-suppressed precontrast images. This can lead to an occasional misdiagnosis by assuming that all the high signal on the postcontrast image is from contrast enhancement,

A   **B**

F<small>IGURE</small> **3-39   Schwannoma.** Coronal T1- *(A)* and T2-weighted *(B)* images of an ankle in a young woman with a painful mass show a homogeneous mass that seems to emanate from the joint itself, suggesting an atypical ganglion. IV contrast should have been administered to determine if this were a solid or a cystic mass. At surgery, this was found to be a solid tumor, a benign schwannoma.

thereby making the call of a solid mass. A fluid collection can sometimes appear to enhance on the postcontrast images simply as a result of the fat suppression (Fig. 3-40). When comparing precontrast and postcontrast images, it is important to not change anything else, or you won't know for sure what's causing the increased signal in the mass.

There is no good reason to fat-suppress the postcontrast images—it simply makes for prettier pictures, but at the expense of an occasional misdiagnosis. If you must fat-suppress the postcontrast images, you must also fat-suppress the precontrast images so that you have only changed one variable.

FIGURE 3-40 **Hemorrhagic cyst.** A 61-year-old man presented with a mass on his thigh that was revealed to be of intermediate signal on an axial T1-weighted image (*A, arrow*). A coronal T2-weighted image shows marked high signal, which is homogeneous. Is this solid or cystic? A coronal T1-weighted image with fat suppression was performed after administration of gadolinium (*C*), which shows apparent diffuse enhancement indicating this is a solid mass. However, the increased signal cannot reliably be attributed to enhancement from the gadolinium because fat suppression was applied, which, in some instances, can make a mass appear brighter simply because of its relatively higher signal compared with the muscles. Notice on the T1 image in *A* that the mass is higher in signal than the muscles; therefore, when fat suppression is applied, the next highest signal structure is the mass. Scaling the image then makes it appear bright, which can be misinterpreted as secondary to contrast enhancement. This was incorrectly called a solid tumor, and at surgery was found to be a hemorrhagic cyst.

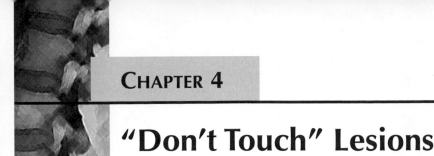

CHAPTER 4

"Don't Touch" Lesions

Skeletal "don't touch" lesions are those processes that are so radiographically characteristic that a biopsy or additional diagnostic tests are unnecessary. Not only does the biopsy result in unnecessary morbidity and cost, but, in some instances, a biopsy also can be frankly misleading and lead to additional unnecessary surgery.

Most of our radiology training teaches us to give a differential diagnosis of a lesion, leaving it up to the clinician to decide between the various entities. For the "don't touch" lesions, however, a differential list is inappropriate, because that often makes the next step on the decision tree a biopsy. Because a biopsy of these lesions is not required for a final diagnosis, a radiologic diagnosis should be made without a list of differential possibilities. "Don't touch" lesions can be classified into three categories: (1) posttraumatic lesions, (2) normal variants, and (3) lesions that are real but obviously benign.

POSTTRAUMATIC LESIONS

Myositis ossificans is an example of a lesion on which a biopsy should not be performed because its aggressive histologic appearance can often mimic a sarcoma. Unfortunately, radical surgery has been performed on the basis of the histologic appearance of myositis ossificans when the radiologic appearance was diagnostic. The typical radiologic appearance of myositis ossificans is circumferential calcification with a lucent center (Fig. 4-1). This is often best appreciated on computed tomography (CT) examination (Fig. 4-2). A malignant tumor that mimics myositis ossificans will have an ill-defined periphery and a calcified or ossific center (Fig. 4-3). Periosteal reaction can be seen with myositis ossificans or with a tumor. Occasionally, the peripheral calcification of myositis ossificans can be difficult to appreciate; in such cases, a CT scan should help, or delayed films a

week or two later are recommended. Biopsy should be avoided when myositis ossificans is a clinical consideration. Magnetic resonance imaging (MRI) in myositis ossificans can be misleading because the peripheral calcification may not be conspicuous and often has marked soft tissue edema surrounding it (Fig. 4-4).

Another posttraumatic entity on which a biopsy can be misleading is an avulsion injury. These injuries can have an aggressive radiographic appearance, but because of their characteristic location at insertion sites (e.g., anteroinferior iliac spine or ischial tuberosity), they should be recognized as benign (Figs. 4-5 and 4-6). Again, delayed films of several weeks will usually allow the problem case to become more radiographically and clinically clear. Biopsy can lead to the mistaken diagnosis of a sarcoma, and should therefore be avoided. Any area that is undergoing healing can have a high nuclear–chromatin ratio and a high mitotic figure count, thereby occasionally simulating a malignancy.

A cortical desmoid is a process considered by many to be an avulsion off the medial supracondylar ridge of the distal femur. It occasionally simulates an aggressive lesion radiographically, and on biopsy can look malignant.[1] In many instances, biopsy has led to amputation for this benign, radiographically characteristic lesion (Figs. 4-7 to 4-9). Cortical desmoids occur only on the posteromedial epicondyle of the femur. They may or may not be associated with pain and can have increased radionuclide uptake on bone scan. They may or may not exhibit periosteal new bone and usually occur in young people. Biopsy should be avoided in all cases. They are often seen as incidental findings on MRI and have a characteristic appearance (Fig. 4-10).

Trauma can lead to large, cystic geodes or subchondral cysts near joints that can be mistaken for

A   **B**

FIGURE 4-1   **Myositis ossificans.** *A,* A plain film of the femur in this patient, who presented with a soft tissue mass, shows a calcific density adjacent to the posterior cortex of the femur that is calcified primarily in its periphery. From seeing the plain film alone, it should not be difficult to definitely say that this is peripheral, circumferential calcification; however, the CT scan shown in *(B)* is helpful in showing that the calcification is unequivocally peripheral. This is virtually diagnostic of myositis ossificans.

A   **B**

FIGURE 4-2   **Myositis ossificans.** *A,* Hazy calcification is seen adjacent to the humeral shaft, with underlying periosteal reaction noted. It is difficult to ascertain whether the calcification is circumferential. *B,* A CT scan through this mass shows that the calcification is unequivocally circumferential, making the diagnosis of myositis ossificans a certainty.

FIGURE 4-3 **Osteogenic sarcoma.** Hazy, ill-defined calcification is seen adjacent to the iliac wing in this patient that can be ascertained from the plain film to definitely not be circumferential. Even though a prior history of trauma was obtained in this case, myositis ossificans is not a consideration with this appearance of calcification. Biopsy showed this to be an osteogenic sarcoma.

other lesions; thus, a biopsy is performed. Although the biopsy specimen is not likely to mimic a malignant process, it is nevertheless avoidable. Because geodes from degenerative disease almost always are associated with additional findings, such as joint space narrowing, sclerosis, and osteophytes, a diagnosis should be made radiographically (Figs. 4-11 and 4-12). However, on occasion, the additional findings are subtle and can be missed (Fig. 4-13). Geodes can also occur in the setting of calcium pyrophosphate dihydrate crystal disease (also known as CPPD or pseudogout), rheumatoid arthritis, and avascular necrosis.[2]

An entity that is often confused with metastatic disease to the spine is discogenic vertebral disease. It can mimic metastatic disease radiographically and clinically, and unless the radiologist is familiar with this process, it can lead to an unnecessary biopsy.[3,4] Discogenic vertebral disease most often is sclerotic and focal (Fig. 4-14). It is adjacent to an end-plate, and the associated disc space should be narrow. Osteophytosis is invariably present. It represents a variant of a Schmorl's node and should not be confused with a metastatic focus. Occasionally it can be lytic or even mixed lytic-sclerotic. The typical clinical setting is a middle-aged woman with chronic low back pain. Old films often confirm the benign nature of this process. In the set-

A   **B**   **C**

FIGURE 4-4 **Myositis ossificans.** *A,* A plain film of the humerus in this 30-year-old man shows a calcific mass adjacent to the diaphysis of the humerus. The calcification is not clearly peripheral in nature, although the central portion is less well mineralized. *B,* An axial T2-weighted image through the mass shows only a high-signal mass without evidence of calcification. *C,* A CT scan through the mass demonstrates the typical peripheral calcification, which is virtually pathognomonic for myositis ossificans.

FIGURE 4-5   **Avulsion injury.** Cortical irregularity (*arrows*) at the ischial tuberosity in this patient with pain over this region raises the question of possible tumor. This is a classic appearance, however, for an avulsion injury from this region, and a biopsy should be avoided.

FIGURE 4-6   **Avulsion injury.** Cortical irregularity with a Codman's triangle of periostitis is seen along the ischial tuberosity. This was at first thought to represent a malignancy. Because of the characteristic location, an avulsion injury was considered and the lesion was observed. It healed without sequelae. (Case courtesy Dr. John Wilson.)

FIGURE 4-7   **Cortical desmoid.** A focal cortical irregularity is seen in the posterior aspect of the femur (*arrow*) with adjacent periostitis noted. Although a tumor such as an early parosteal osteosarcoma could perhaps have this appearance, the location and appearance are characteristic of a cortical desmoid, and a biopsy should not be performed.

FIGURE 4-8 **Cortical desmoid.** Cortical irregularity with periostitis is seen in the posterior distal femur (*arrow*), which is characteristic in location and appearance for a cortical desmoid.

FIGURE 4-9 **Cortical desmoid.** A well-defined cortical defect is seen in the posterior distal femur (*arrow*), which is a common appearance for a fairly well healed cortical desmoid.

ting of disc-space narrowing and osteophytosis, a biopsy of focal sclerosis adjacent to an end-plate should not be performed.

Occasionally, a fracture will be the cause of extensive osteosclerosis and periostitis, which can

mimic a primary bone tumor (Fig. 4-15). Lack of immobilization can result in exuberant callus, which can be misinterpreted as aggressive periostitis or even tumor new bone. A biopsy in such a case might resemble a malignant lesion. Therefore, any case associated with trauma should be carefully reviewed for a fracture.

Another traumatic process that can be misdiagnosed radiologically, leading to inappropriate treatment and morbidity, is a pseudodislocation of the humerus (Figs. 4-16 and 4-17). This results from a fracture with hemarthrosis, which causes distention of the joint and migration of the humeral head inferiorly. An axial or transscapular view shows that it is not anteriorly or posteriorly dislocated (the usual forms of shoulder dislocation) but merely inferiorly displaced. On an anteroposterior view it can mimic a posterior dislocation. Often, attempts are made to "relocate" the humeral head, which are both fruitless (because it is not dislocated) and painful. A fracture is invariably present, and if not seen on the initial films, it should be sought after with additional views. A transscapular or an axillary view is the key to making the diagnosis of a pseudodislocation. With either of these views, the humeral head can be seen to be normally positioned in relation to the glenoid, although it may appear somewhat inferiorly displaced. If necessary, the joint can be aspirated to confirm the presence of a bloody effusion and to show the normal position of the humeral head with no fluid in the joint.[5]

Costochondritis, or Tietze's syndrome, can cause a bulbous swelling of a rib (Fig. 4-18) caused by periostitis, which can mimic a rib lesion. This condition is painful and usually easily diagnosed clinically; however, with a bony lesion seen on radiographs, many clinicians may want a biopsy to rule out a malignant process. This would be a mistake, as with any posttraumatic or rapidly healing lesion, it can be difficult to categorize histologically. Because Tietze's syndrome is a short-lived process, watchful waiting with repeat film in 2 to 3 weeks if the patient's condition has not improved is probably indicated.

NORMAL VARIANTS

Numerous normal variants exist that are often confused with a pathologic process. This is best evidenced by the fact that several of the most popular radiology texts are atlases of normal variants.

A normal variant that has been described in the patella is a lytic defect in the upper outer quadrant called dorsal defect of the patella (Fig. 4-19).[6] It can mimic a focus of infection, osteochondritis dissecans (Fig. 4-20), or a chondroblastoma. It is a normal developmental anomaly, however, and

FIGURE 4-10   Cortical desmoid. *A,* An anteroposterior film of the knee in a child shows a faint lytic lesion *(arrows)* in the medial aspect of the distal femur. Axial T1-*(B)* and T2-weighted *(C)* images through the lesion show a cortically based process *(arrows)* in the medial supracondylar ridge, which is characteristic for a cortical desmoid.

because of its characteristic location, a biopsy of it should not be performed. It is diagnosed on MRI also by its characteristic location, as the signal characteristics are similar to tumor or infection (Fig. 4-21).

Another entity often confused with a lytic pathologic process is a pseudocyst of the humerus

(Fig. 4-22). This is merely an anatomic variant caused by the increased cancellous bone in the region of the greater tuberosity of the humerus, which gives this region a more lucent appearance on radiographs. With hyperemia and disuse caused by rotator cuff problems or any other shoulder disorder, this area of lucency may appear strikingly

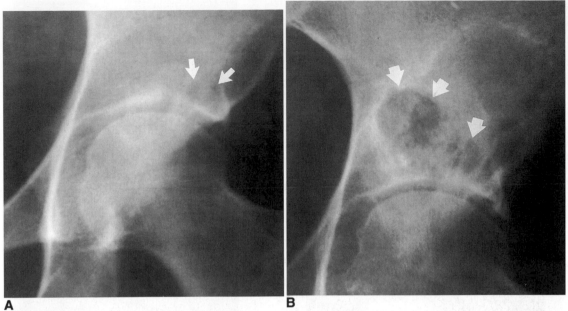

A **B**

FIGURE 4-11 Geode. *A,* A plain film of the hip in this older patient with hip pain shows a lytic lesion in the supraacetabular region *(arrow),* which has a benign appearance. Mild osteoarthritis was believed to be present (when compared with the opposite hip, joint space narrowing and minimal sclerosis were seen); hence, this was believed to be a subchondral cyst or geode. *B,* Several years later, the same hip shows a large lytic lesion *(arrows)* that still appears benign. The osteoarthritis has increased in severity. However, because of the growth of the lesion it was biopsied and found to be a geode.

FIGURE 4-12 Geode. A large cystic lesion was found in the shoulder in this middle-aged weight lifter, and the possibility of a metastatic process was considered. Because the humeral head has sclerosis and osteophytosis, as well as a loose body in the joint *(arrow),* the degenerative disease of the shoulder was diagnosed; this makes the cystic lesion almost certainly a geode or subchondral cyst, which made a biopsy unnecessary.

more lucent and mimic a lytic lesion. Biopsies of many of these lesions have been done mistakenly, and, in several cases, have been repeated (see Fig. 4-22C) after the initial pathology report stated "normal bone—no lesion in specimen." Because of the associated hyperemia from the shoulder disorder (be it rotator cuff or whatever), a bone scan can show increased radionuclide uptake and thus sway the surgeon to do a biopsy of this normal variant. It is radiographically characteristic in its location and appearance, and a biopsy of it should not be done.[7] Although other lesions, such as a chondroblastoma (Fig. 4-23), infection, or even a metastatic focus, could occur in a similar location, they do not have quite the same appearance as a pseudocyst of the humerus.

A normal variant of the cervical spine that may, in fact, be posttraumatic is an os odontoideum.[8] It is an unfused dens that may move anterior to the C-2 body with flexion, and can mimic a fractured dens (Figs. 4-24 and 4-25). Many of these lesions require surgical fixation; some surgeons fuse every case, believing that they are all unstable. Radiologists should recognize that this process is not acute, so as to save the patient from having Crutchfield tongs or a halo applied and from possible immediate surgical intervention. Most cases

A

B

FIGURE 4-13 **Geode.** *A,* A cystic lesion was noted in the femoral head *(arrows)* of a young man with a painful hip. *B,* A CT scan through this area shows the subarticular nature and adjacent sclerosis. The differential diagnosis of infection, eosinophilic granuloma, and chondroblastoma was given. A ring of osteophytes *(open arrowheads)* was noted in retrospect on the plain film *(A)* in the subcapital region, which indicates degenerative disease of the hip. This is an extremely unusual presentation in a healthy 20-year-old man; however, it makes the lytic lesion in the femoral head almost certainly a subchondral cyst or geode. This was an active soccer player who had been playing with pain in his hip for several years after an injury that had caused the degenerative disease. Unfortunately, a biopsy was performed anyway, and a subchondral cyst or geode was confirmed.

A

B

C

FIGURE 4-14 **Discogenic vertebral sclerosis.** *A-C,* These films all show patients with sclerosis on the inferior portion of the L-4 vertebral body associated with minimal osteophytosis and joint space narrowing at the adjacent disc space. This is the classic appearance for discogenic vertebral sclerosis, and a biopsy to rule out metastatic disease should not be performed.

A   **B**

Figure 4-15   Fracture mimicking osteosarcoma. A, This 16-year-old had experienced pain around the knee for 2 weeks before these radiographs were taken. The knee films showed diffuse sclerosis and extensive periostitis about the distal femur, which was believed to be characteristic for an osteogenic sarcoma. The periosteal reaction, however, was believed to be much too thick, dense, and wavy to represent malignant type of periostitis. B, A small offset of the epiphysis can be seen (arrow), which indicates an epiphyseal slippage consistent with a Salter epiphyseal fracture. The patient had fallen off his bicycle and fractured his femur, yet continued to be active. The lack of immobility caused exuberant periostitis or callus with a large amount of reactive sclerosis, all of which mimicked an osteogenic sarcoma.

A   **B**

Figure 4-16   Pseudodislocation of the shoulder. A, This patient experienced trauma to the shoulder, with resultant pain and immobility, and was thought to have a dislocation of the shoulder after the anteroposterior film was seen. The humeral head is inferiorly placed in relation to the glenoid; however, this is not the characteristic location of an anterior or posterior dislocation. B, The transscapular view shows the humeral head to be situated normally over the glenoid without anterior or posterior dislocation. These findings are characteristic for a pseudodislocation caused by hemarthrosis, or blood in the joint, which allows the shoulder to be subluxed rather than dislocated. Aspiration of the blood will result in the humeral head returning to its normal position in relation to the glenoid; however, this is not usually necessary. When a pseudodislocation is seen, as in this example, search for an occult fracture should ensue. In this case as seen on A a fracture (arrow) was initially missed.

are seen after trauma, and if no neurologic deficits are present, these patients can be seen electively and spared the horrors and morbidity associated with treatment of the acutely fractured cervical spine. The radiologic signs for recognizing an os odontoideum are the smooth, often well-corticated inferior border of the dens and the hypertrophied, densely corticated anterior arch of C-1. This latter finding presumably represents compensatory hypertrophy and indicates a long-standing condition.[9]

Although unusual, osteopoikilosis, a benign familial process of multiple bone islands or small areas of osteosclerosis, has caused confusion by its similarity to metastatic disease (Fig. 4-26). Ordinarily osteopoikilosis has such a characteristic appearance that it will not be mistaken for another entity, and the predominance of sclerotic foci near the epiphyses should help to differentiate it from metastatic disease (Fig. 4-27).

FIGURE 4-17 **Pseudodislocation of the shoulder.** The humeral head is inferiorly placed in relation to the glenoid. This is the characteristic location when a hemarthrosis is present. A minimally displaced fracture of the neck of the humerus with avulsion of the greater tuberosity has occurred, causing the hemarthrosis.

A   **B**

FIGURE 4-18 **Costochondritis.** *A,* A young male patient with point tenderness over the anterior chest wall had a chest radiograph that revealed a nodular density *(arrow)* that appeared attached to the second rib. *B,* Tomograms of this area show a nodular density with speckled calcification at the distal end of the rib, which was thought to possibly represent an osteochondroma. Any chondroid lesion that is painful should be suspicious for malignant degeneration, and a biopsy was planned for this patient. The clinical findings, however, were classic for costochondritis or Tietze's syndrome, which rapidly cleared; therefore, the biopsy was canceled. Costochondritis can cause periostitis and bulbous swelling of the ribs, as in this example, and a biopsy should not be performed.

A   **B**

FIGURE 4-19   **Dorsal defect of the patella.** A lytic defect in the upper outer quadrant of the patella (*A*) was seen in this patient (*arrows*), which is characteristic for a normal variant called dorsal defect of the patella. It occurs only in the upper outer quadrant and should be asymptomatic. It lies adjacent to the articular surface as shown on the sunrise view (*B*).

A   **B**

FIGURE 4-20   **Osteochondritis dissecans of the patella.** *A* and *B,* A defect in the articular surface of the patella (*arrows*) is seen in this patient. It is centrally placed rather than in the upper outer quadrant. Because of its location, a dorsal defect of the patella is not a consideration. This was osteochondritis dissecans, which is unusual in the patella.

FIGURE 4-21   **MR images of dorsal defect of the patella.** *A,* T1- and *(B)* T2-weighted axial MR images through the patella in a patient with a lytic lesion in the upper outer quadrant of the patella shows low signal on the T1 image, which is high signal on T2. This is a characteristic appearance for a dorsal defect of the patella because of its location.

OBVIOUSLY BENIGN LESIONS

Biopsies are frequently performed on some lesions that should be recognized radiographically as benign and left alone. These are lesions that should be diagnosed by the radiologist, not the pathologist. Listing a differential in such cases often spurs the surgeon to a biopsy, when in fact no biopsy should be necessary.

Perhaps the most commonly encountered lesion in this category is the nonossifying fibroma (NOF). It is identical to a fibrous cortical defect, but the term is usually reserved for defects larger than 2 cm. NOFs are, classically, lytic lesions that are located in the cortex of the metaphysis of a long bone that have a well-defined, often sclerotic, scalloped border with slight cortical expansion (Fig. 4-28) (see also Chapter 2). They are almost

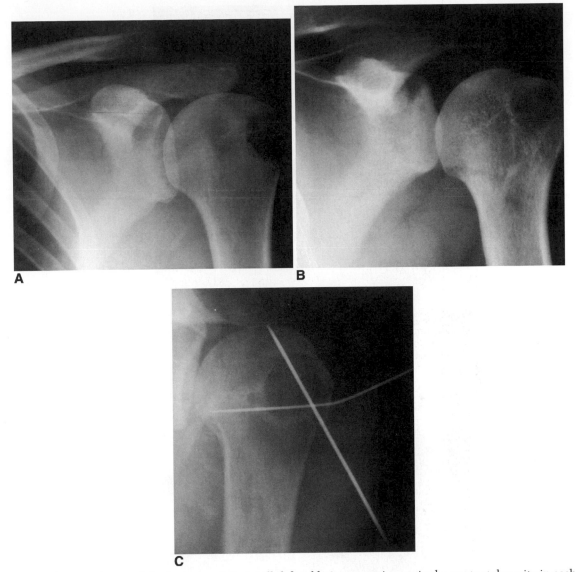

FIGURE 4-22 **Pseudocyst of the humerus.** *A-C,* A well-defined lytic process is seen in the greater tuberosity in each of these examples. In each case it was believed to represent a lytic lesion. These patients were all symptomatic, and several had increased radionuclide uptake on isotope bone scan. The location and appearance, however, are characteristic for a pseudocyst of the humerus, which merely represents decreased cortical bone in this region. This becomes more pronounced when pain in the shoulder is present and hyperemia or disuse osteoporosis occurs. Biopsies of several of these examples were performed, and a biopsy was repeated in the example in *C* when the first biopsy was reported as "normal bone" and the surgeons assumed that they had missed the lesion.

exclusively found in patients younger than 30 years, suggesting that the natural history of the lesion is involution. As they involute, they fill in with new bone (Fig. 4-29); hence, they can have some increased radionuclide activity on bone scans. They are most often mistaken for an area of infection, eosinophilic granuloma, or aneurysmal bone cyst. NOFs are asymptomatic and have never been reported to be associated with malignant degeneration. Occasionally, a pathologic fracture

can occur through these lesions, but most surgeons do not advocate prophylactic curettage to prevent fracture, as with unicameral bone cysts. NOFs can be quite large, but invariably have a benign appearance (Fig. 4-30), and biopsy should be avoided. The asymptomatic nature is imperative to help distinguish them from most of the other lesions in the differential, thereby precluding even giving a differential diagnosis. On occasion, they are found to be multiple (Fig. 4-31), yet each

FIGURE 4-23 **Chondroblastoma.** A well-defined lesion in the greater tuberosity of the humerus that has a sclerotic margin is easily distinguished from the prior examples of pseudocyst of the humerus. This was found to be a chondroblastoma.

A   **B**

FIGURE 4-24 **Os odontoideum.** Flexion (A) and extension (B) views show that the anterior arch (A) of the C-1 vertebrae has moved markedly anterior in relation to the body of C-2 in flexion. The odontoid or dens is difficult to see but appears to be separated from the body of C-2. Because of the smooth borders of the separated dens and because of the cortical hypertrophy of the anterior arch of C-1, this can safely be called an os odontoideum, which is a congenital or long-standing post-traumatic abnormality rather than an acute fracture. Obviously, these patients should have no neurologic problems, yet in many instances the lesions are still believed to be unstable and are surgically fused. Surgery, if indicated, can be done on an elective basis.

A   **B**

FIGURE 4-25   Os odontoideum. Extension (A) and flexion (B) show extreme motion of the anterior arch (A) of C-1 as compared with the C-2 vertebral body. The dens is difficult to find in this example but is certainly not attached to the C-2 body. Again, the smooth margins where the dens should be attached and the cortical hypertrophy of the anterior arch of C-1 make this a congenital or long-standing process consistent with an os odontoideum rather than an acute fracture.

A   **B**

C   **D**

FIGURE 4-26   Diffuse metastatic disease mimicking osteopoikilosis. A,B, A CT scan through the pelvis and hips shows diffuse sclerotic foci consistent with metastatic disease. One examiner believed that this might represent the sclerotic foci of osteopoikilosis, however, which is a benign familial process. C, An anteroposterior view of the pelvis shows a similar appearance; however, a destructive lytic lesion is seen in the right proximal femur, which makes metastatic disease more likely. This patient had metastatic prostate carcinoma. Compare this with D in a patient with known osteopoikilosis and it is easy to see how the two entities can be confused. Clinical history is vital in the distinction.

FIGURE 4-27 **Osteopoikilosis.** A more typical example of osteopoikilosis is shown in this example, in which the sclerotic foci are predominantly around the joints rather than diffusely spread throughout the bones.

A

FIGURE 4-28 **Nonossifying fibroma.** A well-defined, slightly expansile lytic lesion is seen in a long bone, which is characteristic for a nonossifying fibroma. Unfortunately, a biopsy of the lesion was performed, and the diagnosis was surgically confirmed.

B

FIGURE 4-29 **Healing nonossifying fibroma.** *A,* A minimally sclerotic, slightly expansile process is seen in the posterior proximal tibia *(arrows).* This was believed by the surgeons to represent a focus of infection or an osteoid osteoma even though the patient was asymptomatic. This is a characteristic appearance for a disappearing or healing nonossifying fibroma. The postsurgical appearance, which went on to a pathologic fracture, is shown in *B.* Surgery confirmed a nonossifying fibroma.

A   **B**

FIGURE 4-30   **Nonossifying fibroma.** *A* and *B,* This well-defined, minimally expansile lytic lesion of the proximal tibia is characteristic for a nonossifying fibroma. It was believed by several radiologists to be a giant cell tumor; however, it has a sclerotic border and does not abut the tibial articular surface. Even though the patient was asymptomatic, a biopsy was performed and the diagnosis of a nonossifying fibroma was confirmed. (Case courtesy Dr. Larry Yeager.)

A   **B**

FIGURE 4-31   **Multiple nonossifying fibromas.** Multiple well-defined lytic lesions *(arrows)* are seen around the knees in this patient on the anteroposterior *(A)* and lateral *(B)* views, each of which is characteristic for a nonossifying fibroma.

lesion is so characteristic that they should be easily diagnosed.

Bone islands are not a radiographic dilemma when they are 1 cm or less. Occasionally, however, they grow to golf ball size and mimic sclerotic metastases (Fig. 4-32). They are always asymptomatic. Radiographically, two signs can be found to help distinguish giant bone islands from metastases. First, bone islands usually are oblong, with their long axis in the axis of stress on the bone (e.g., in a long bone they align themselves along the axis of the diaphysis). Second, the margins of a bone island, if examined closely, will show bony trabeculae extending from the lesion into the normal bone in a spiculated fashion[10] (see Chapter 2). This is characteristic of a bone island and is helpful in differentiating it from more aggressive processes.

Unicameral bone cysts are often prophylactically packed so as to prevent fracture with subsequent deformity. When these cysts occur in the calcaneus, however, they should be left alone. They always occur in the anteroinferior portion of the calcaneus (Fig. 4-33), an area that does not receive undue stress. In fact, a pseudotumor of the calcaneus in the identical position is seen because of the absence of stress and resulting atrophy of bony trabeculae (Fig. 4-34). Calcaneal unicameral

bone cysts are asymptomatic, only rarely fracture, and should not suffer the same fate as their counterparts in long bones. Calcaneal unicameral bone cysts seem to involute at a slower rate than those in long bones; hence, they can be seen in patients older than 30 years. Also, as they involute, they occasionally undergo "lipidization," which is fatty infiltration. If they are imaged or if a biopsy is performed during this stage, they get mistakenly diagnosed as an intraosseous lipoma. This is why many authors have called calcaneal unicameral bone cysts lipomas. Annually, around radiology oral boards time, residents ask me to explain why some texts refer to these lesions as unicameral bone cysts and others call them lipomas. In fact, they are all unicameral bone cysts. Many benign fibro-osseous lesions throughout the skeleton involute with fatty infiltration and get mistakenly called intraosseous lipomas.

Early in the course of its development a bone infarct can have a patchy or a mixed lytic-sclerotic pattern, or even resemble a permeative process (Figs. 4-35 and 4-36). In a patient with bone pain and a permeative bone lesion, many aggressive disorders head the differential list and a biopsy soon ensues. If this process can be noted to be multiple and in the diametaphyseal region of a long bone, especially if the patient has an underlying

A   **B**

FIGURE 4-32   **Giant bone island.** *A,* A large sclerotic focus is seen in the right iliac wing, which was thought to possibly represent an area of metastasis. *B,* Old films from 5 years earlier were obtained, which showed a similar but much smaller process. This is characteristic for a growing bone island. Note in *A* how the lesion is somewhat spherical or oblong in the lines of trabecular stress, which is characteristic of a bone island.

FIGURE 4-33 **Unicameral bone cyst.** A well-defined lytic lesion on the anteroinferior portion of the calcaneus, as in this example, is virtually pathognomonic for a unicameral bone cyst or simple bone cyst. Because this is an area of diminished stress, it is thought not to be necessary to prophylactically curettage and pack this lesion in an effort to avoid a pathologic bone fracture, which is often done in the femur and humerus with unicameral bone cysts.

FIGURE 4-34 **Pseudocyst of the calcaneus.** An area of radiolucency is seen in the anteroinferior portion of the calcaneus that is similar to the example in Figure 4-33 but is not as well defined. This is a pseudocyst similar to the pseudocyst of the humerus that results from diminished stress through this region.

FIGURE 4-35 **Early bone infarct.** Patchy demineralization is seen in the distal femur and proximal tibia in this patient with systemic lupus erythematosus. The opposite leg was similarly involved. This is characteristic for early bone infarcts and should not be confused with infection or metastatic disease.

disorder such as sickle cell anemia or systemic lupus erythematosus, areas of early bone infarction should be considered. In several instances, the MRI appearance of an infarct has saved patients from biopsy when the plain films were equivocal (Fig. 4-37).[11]

A commonly encountered lytic lesion on the lateral aspect of the femoral neck was first described by Michael Pitt as a synovial herniation pit.[12] It has taken on the appropriate eponym of a "Pitt's pit." It is believed to be caused by surface erosion of the synovium and soft tissues around the hip, but its exact cause is unknown. It has a characteristic plain film and MRI appearance primarily because of its location and benign appearance (Fig. 4-38).

CONCLUSION

These are but a few of the many examples in skeletal radiology in which the well-trained radiologist can be of invaluable assistance to the clinician and the patient by helping to avert a needless biopsy. Dozens of other examples are nicely shown in normal variant textbooks, which are widely available. Because of the potential harm in performing a needless biopsy, these examples are stressed. When these lesions are encountered by the radiologist, a differential diagnosis should not be offered, because it will merely lead the surgeon to a biopsy in an attempt to reach a diagnosis. A biopsy in many of these entities not only is unnecessary, but also can be misleading.

FIGURE 4-36   **Bone infarct.** A mixed lytic-sclerotic process is seen in the distal femurs and proximal tibias bilaterally in this patient with systemic lupus erythematosus. Because of pain in these regions, a biopsy was performed, and bone infarct was confirmed. With this characteristic location and this appearance, even though suggestive of a more aggressive process, a biopsy of these lesions should not be performed.

A   **B**

FIGURE 4-37   **Bone infarct.** *A*, A plain film of the knee shows faint patchy sclerosis in the proximal tibia that was at first thought to be infection or malignancy. *B*, MRI shows the characteristic serpiginous border seen with bone infarct. MRI, on occasion, can better characterize the ill-defined early bone infarct, as in this example.

FIGURE 4-38 **Pitt's pit.** *A,* A plain film of the left hip shows a well-defined lytic lesion in the lateral aspect of the femoral neck. It has a sclerotic border. This is a characteristic appearance of a synovial herniation pit, also called a Pitt's pit. *B,* T1- and *(C)* T2-weighted MR axial images through the hips show bilateral lesions with low-signal T1 and high-signal T2, which is typical for Pitt's pits.

REFERENCES

1. Barnes G, Gwinn J: Distal irregularities of the femur simulating malignancy. Am J Roentgenol Radium Ther Nucl Med 1974;122:180-185.
2. Resnick D, Niwayama G, Coutts RD: Subchondral cysts (geodes) in arthritic disorders: Pathologic and radiographic appearance of the hip joint. AJR Am J Roentgenol 1977;128:799-806.
3. Martel W, Seeger FJ, Wicks JD, et al: Traumatic lesions of the discovertebral junction in the lumbar spine. Am J Roentgenol 1976;127:457-464.
4. Lipson S: Discogenic vertebral sclerosis with calcified disc. N Engl J Med 1991;325:794-799.
5. Helms C, Richmond B, Sims R: Pseudodislocation of the shoulder: A sign of an occult fracture. Emerg Med 1986;18:237-241.

6. Goergen TG, Resnick D, Greenway G, et al: Dorsal defect of the patella (DDP): A characteristic radiographic lesion. Radiology 1979;130:333-336.

7. Helms C: Pseudocyst of the humerus. AJR 1979; 131:287-292.

8. Minderhoud JM, Braakman R, Penning L: Os odontoideum: Clinical, radiological and therapeutic aspects. J Neurol Sci 1969;8:521-544.

9. Holt RG, Helms CA, Munk PL, Gillespy T III: Hypertrophy of C-1 anterior arch: Useful sign to distinguish os odontoideum from acute dens fracture. Radiology 1989;173:207-209.

10. Onitsuka H: Roentgenologic aspects of bone islands. Radiology 1977;124:607-612.

11. Munk PL, Helms CA, Holt RG: Immature bone infarcts: Findings on plain radiographs and MR scans. AJR 1989;152(3):547-549.

12. Pitt M, Graham A, Shipman J, Birkby W: Herniation pit of the femoral neck. AJR 1982;138:1115-1121.

CHAPTER 5

Trauma

Radiology of trauma to the skeletal system is such a large topic that entire volumes have been devoted to it. Lee Rogers[1] has written the definitive work in his excellent book entitled *Radiology of Skeletal Trauma,* and Jack and William Harris'[2] outstanding book *Radiology of Emergency Medicine* is a must read for anyone dealing with a large emergency department population. The leading orthopedic treatise on fractures is Rockwood and Green's[3] multivolume text. This chapter is merely an overview of selected cases that residents and medical students should be exposed to that can be studied in greater detail by referring to the textbooks mentioned above.

Before starting with specific examples, the uninitiated or neophyte radiologist should keep a few key points in mind concerning radiology of trauma. First, have a high index of suspicion. Every radiologist in the world has missed fractures on radiographs because they were not sufficiently attuned to the fact that a fracture might be present. Often, the history is either nonexistent or misleading, and the anatomic area of concern is therefore overlooked. When in doubt, examine the patient! Orthopedic surgeons seldom miss seeing fractures on radiographs because they have examined the patient, they know where the patient hurts, and they have a high index of suspicion. Second, always get two radiographs at 90 degrees to each other in every trauma case. A high percentage of fractures are seen only on one view (the anteroposterior [AP] or the lateral) and will therefore be missed unless two views are routinely obtained. Third, once a fracture is identified, don't forget to look at the rest of the film. About 10% of all cases have a second finding that often is as significant as, or even more significant than, the initial finding. Many fractures have associated dislocation, foreign bodies, or additional fractures, so be sure to examine the entire film.

SPINE

Examination of the Cervical Spine

The cervical spine is one of the most commonly x-rayed parts of the body in a busy emergency department and can present the most difficulty in interpretation. Usually a cross-table lateral of the cervical spine (C-spine) is obtained first, so as not to unduly move the patient who might have a cervical fracture. If results of the lateral C-spine appear normal, the remainder of the C-spine series, which may include flexion and extension views (if the patient can cooperate), is obtained.

What do you look for on the lateral C-spine? First, make certain that all seven cervical vertebral bodies can be visualized. A large number of fractures are missed because the shoulders obscure the lower C-spine levels (Fig. 5-1). If the entire cervical spine is not visualized, repeat the film with the shoulders lowered.

What constitutes complete visualization of the cervical spine? Many radiologists insist on seeing the top of the T-1 vertebral body on the lateral view, whereas others will pass a C-spine lateral film if it includes any of the C-7 body. Most texts say the lateral view should show "C-1 through C-7." What does "through C-7" mean? I have no idea, but I was trained to accept a lateral C-spine film that included *any* of the C-7 body. It can be difficult to image the T-1 vertebral body in the majority of cases; therefore, I feel it is adequate to accept a lateral C-spine film with *any* of the C-7 vertebral body visible if the report includes the disclaimer that the C-7 to T-1 disc space is not seen and clinical correlation must be obtained to warrant additional films or a CT scan of that area. In fact, this is a moot point in many practices which routinely acquire CT scans throughout the C-spine instead of plain films. Complete

CT evaluation of the cervical spine will probably evolve to be the standard of care, but it is not yet widely accepted as the normal routine.

Next, evaluate five parallel (more or less) lines for stepoff or discontinuity as follows (Fig. 5-2*A* and *B*):

Line 1 is in the prevertebral soft tissue. It extends down the posterior aspect of the airway; it should be several millimeters from the first three or four vertebral bodies and then move farther away at the laryngeal cartilage; it should be less than one vertebral body width from the anterior vertebral bodies from C-3 or C-4 to C-7; and it should be smooth in its contour.

Line 2 follows the anterior vertebral bodies and should be smooth and uninterrupted. Anterior osteophytes can encroach on this line and extend beyond it, and should therefore be ignored in drawing this line. Interruption of the anterior vertebral body line is a sign of a serious injury (see Fig. 5-1*B*).

Line 3 is similar to the anterior vertebral body line (line 2) except that it connects the posterior vertebral bodies. Like line 2, it should be smooth and uninterrupted; any disruption signifies a serious injury.

Line 4, called the spinolaminar line, connects the posterior junction of the lamina with the spinous processes. The spinal cord lies between lines 3 and 4; therefore, any offset of either of these lines could mean that a bony structure is impinging on the cord. Severe neurologic deficits can result from very little force against the cord, and any bony structure lying on the cord must be recognized as soon as possible.

Line 5 is not really a line so much as a collection of points—the tips of the spinous processes. The spinous processes are quite variable in size and appearance, although C-7 usually has the largest. A fracture of one of the spinous processes, by itself, is not a serious injury, but it occasionally heralds other, more serious injuries. Also, who wants to

A   **B**

FIGURE 5-1 **Shoulders obscuring C-7.** This patient came to the emergency department after being injured as a result of diving into a shallow swimming pool. He had neck pain but no neurologic deficits. The initial radiograph obtained of the cervical spine (C-spine) (*A*) was interpreted as being within normal limits. However, because of high-riding shoulders only five cervical vertebrae are visible. A repeat examination (*B*) with the shoulders lowered reveals a dislocation of C-5 on C-6. To visualize C-7 the shoulders were lowered even further. The C-7 vertebral body must be visualized on every lateral C-spine examination in a trauma setting.

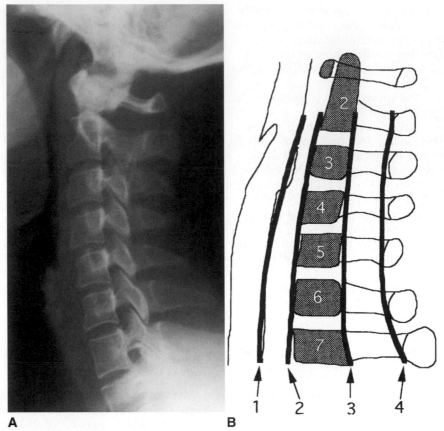

A   **B**

FIGURE 5-2 **Normal lateral cervical spine.** *A,* Lateral radiograph of a normal cervical spine. *B,* Diagrammatic representation of a lateral cervical spine (C-spine) showing four parallel lines that should be observed in every lateral C-spine examination. Line 1 is the soft tissue line that is closely applied to the posterior border of the airway through the first four or five vertebral body segments and then widens around the laryngeal cartilage and runs parallel to the remainder of the cervical vertebrae. Line 2 demarcates the anterior border of the cervical vertebral bodies. Line 3 is the posterior border of the cervical vertebral bodies. Line 4, called the spinolaminar line, is drawn by connecting the junction of the lamina at the spinal process. It represents the posterior extent of the central canal, which contains the spinal cord itself. These lines should generally be smooth and parallel, with no abrupt stepoff.

miss a fractured spinous process, however innocuous, and then have the patient (after visiting another doctor) proclaim that you didn't see his or her "broken neck" on the radiograph?

After visually inspecting these five lines on the lateral C-spine, then inspect the C1-2 area a little more closely. Make certain that the anterior arch of C-1 is no greater than 2.5 mm from the dens (Fig. 5-3*A* and *B*). Any greater separation than this (except in children, in whom up to 5.0 mm is normal) is suspicious for disruption of the transverse ligament between C-1 and C-2 (Fig. 5-4*A* and *B*).

The disc spaces are examined next to see that there is no inordinate widening or narrowing, either of which could indicate an acute traumatic injury. If a disc space is narrowed, it will usually be secondary to degenerative disease. Make certain that associated osteophytosis and sclerosis are present, however, before assuming the narrowing is caused by degenerative disease.

An examination of the lateral C-spine as described earlier can be done in less than 1 minute. If this view is normal, then the remainder of the examination can be completed, including flexion and extension views. It is imperative that the patient initiate the flexion and extension without help from the technician or anyone else. A patient, if conscious and semialert, will not injure himself with voluntary flexion and extension and will have muscle guarding, preventing motion, if an injury is present. Even gentle pressure to aid in flexion or extension can cause severe injury if a fracture or dislocation is present.

I would like to stress the importance of learning to look at lateral spine films with anterior facing either right or left. Many radiologists can only interpret images facing one way, and become almost unable to function if the films are not placed on the view box in their preferred orientation. This is fine if they can control the film; however, in

FIGURE 5-3 Normal C1-2. A lateral radiograph (A) and drawing (B) of the upper cervical spine, showing the normal distance of the anterior arch of C-1 to be less than 2.5 mm from the odontoid process of C-2 (*arrows*).

meetings where slides are shown, in books and journals, and on boards, they cannot turn the film to their liking. Get used to viewing lateral spine films (lateral chest films, too) in either anterior left or right orientation or you will find yourself at a disadvantage in many situations.

Examples of Fractures, Dislocations, and Other Abnormalities

A blow to the top of the head, such as when an object falls directly on the apex of the skull, can cause the lateral masses of C-1 to slide apart,

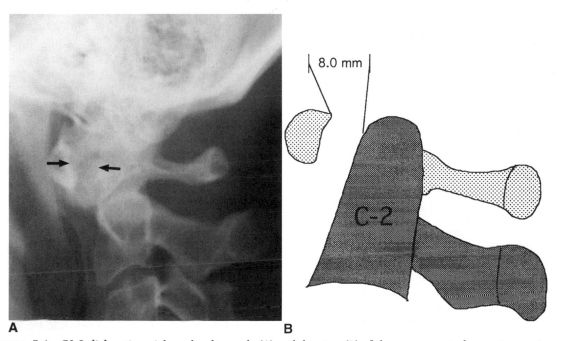

FIGURE 5-4 C1-2 dislocation. A lateral radiograph (A) and drawing (B) of the upper cervical spine in a patient with trauma to the neck, which shows that the anterior arch of C-1 is 8 mm anterior to the odontoid process of C-2 (*arrows*). This is diagnostic of a dislocation of C-1 on C-2 and indicates rupture of the transverse ligaments, which normally hold these vertebral segments together.

A   **B**

FIGURE 5-5   **Jefferson's fracture.** An AP open-mouth odontoid view *(A)* is suspicious for the lateral masses of C-1 being laterally displaced. However, because of overlying structures, this displacement is difficult to appreciate. Therefore, a CT examination *(B)* was obtained, which shows multiple fracture sites in the C-1 ring *(arrows)*. This is called a Jefferson's fracture. CT is routinely used in spinal trauma because of the obvious shortcomings of plain films.

splitting the bony ring of C-1. This is called a *Jefferson's fracture* (Fig. 5-5). It nicely illustrates how a bony ring will not break in just one place, but must break in several places. This rule is seldom violated. All of the vertebral rings, when fractured, must fracture in two or more places. The bony rings of the pelvis behave the same way. If you see only one fracture on the radiograph, you're certainly missing at least one more. CT examination is excellent at demonstrating the complete bony ring of C-1 and shows the fractures, as well as any associated soft tissue mass, much better than plain films. In diagnosing a Jefferson's fracture on plain film, the lateral masses of C-1 must extend beyond the margins of the C-2 body (see Fig. 5-5A). Just seeing asymmetry of the spaces on either side of the dens is not enough to make the diagnosis, because these spaces can be normally asymmetric with rotation or with rotatory fixation of the atlantoaxial joint.

What is *rotatory fixation of the atlantoaxial joint?* This is a somewhat controversial, little understood process in which the atlantoaxial joint becomes fixed and the C-1 and C-2 bodies move en masse instead of rotating on each other. This condition is easily diagnosed with open-mouth odontoid views. In the normal odontoid view the spaces lateral to the dens (odontoid) are equal. With rotation of the head to the left the space on the left widens, and with rotation to the right the space on the right widens. With rotatory fixation, one of the spaces is wider than the other and stays wider even with rotation of the head to the opposite side (Fig. 5-6). By itself, this is a relatively innocuous malady that is usually treated with a soft cervical collar, gentle traction, or both. It is, however, occasionally asso-

ciated with disruption of the transverse ligaments at C1-2, and is then a serious problem. Rotatory fixation usually presents spontaneously or after mild trauma, such as that caused by sleeping in an unusual position.

Another relatively innocuous injury is a fracture of the C-6 or C-7 spinous process, called a *clay-shoveler's fracture.* Supposedly workers shoveling sticky clay in Australia (I've also read England and North Carolina—this is a vital distinction and some future researcher can perhaps straighten out this confusion) would toss the shovelfuls of clay over their shoulders; once in a while the clay would stick to the shovel, causing the ligaments attached to the spinous processes (supraspinous ligaments) to undergo a tremendous force, pulling on the spinous process and avulsing it. This fracture can occur at any of the lower cervical spinous processes (Fig. 5-7).

A *hangman's fracture* is an unstable, serious fracture of the upper cervical spine that is caused by hyperextension and distraction (such as hitting one's head on a dashboard). This is a fracture of the posterior elements of C-2 and, usually, displacement of the C-2 body anterior to C-3 (Fig. 5-8). Patients with this type of fracture actually do better than one might think. They often escape neurologic impairment because of the fractured posterior elements of C-2, which, in effect, cause a decompression and take pressure off the injured area. This is a simplistic explanation for a complex entity, but it seems to be a reasonable answer to why these patients often fare well.

Severe flexion of the cervical spine can cause a disruption of the posterior ligaments and anterior compression of a vertebral body. This is called a

A   **B**

C

FIGURE 5-6   **Rotatory fixation of the atlantoaxial joint.** This patient came to the emergency department with pain and decreased motion in the cervical spine. An AP open-mouth odontoid view *(A)* shows that the space on the left side of the odontoid between the odontoid and the lateral mass of C-1 *(arrows)* is wider than the corresponding space on the right side. This is often caused by rotation. Therefore, open-mouth odontoid views with right and left obliquities were obtained. Rotation of the patient's head to the left *(B)* causes the space on the left side of the odontoid process *(arrows)* to be wider than that on the right, which is appropriate. However, when the patient turns to the right *(C)*, the space on the right *(arrows)* does not get wider than the space on the left. This is diagnostic of rotatory fixation of the atlantoaxial joint.

flexion "teardrop" fracture (Fig. 5-9). A teardrop fracture is usually associated with spinal cord injury, often from the posterior portion of the vertebral body being displaced into the central canal.

If severe enough, and if associated with some rotation, the apophyseal joint ligaments will rupture and the facet joints dislocate and then override. This can result in locking of the facets in an overriding position, which in effect causes some stabilization to protect against further injury. This condition is called *unilateral locked facets* (Figs. 5-10 and 5-11), but, occasionally, it occurs bilat-

erally. When unilateral, the more inferior vertebral body is usually rotated, giving it a shorter AP length on a lateral film, which is a clue to the diagnosis (see Fig. 5-11).

A "seat belt injury" is seen secondary to hyperflexion at the waist (as occurs in a car accident while the person is restrained by a lap belt). This causes distraction of the posterior elements and ligaments and anterior compression of the vertebral body. It usually involves the L1 or L2 level. Several variations of this injury can occur: a fracture of the posterior body is called a *Smith's*

FIGURE 5-7 **Clay-shoveler's fracture.** A nondisplaced fracture of the C-7 spinous process (*arrow*) is noted, which is diagnostic of a clay-shoveler's fracture.

fracture, and a fracture through the spinous process is called a *Chance fracture.* Horizontal fractures of the pedicles, laminae, and transverse processes can also occur (Fig. 5-12).

A somewhat controversial spinal abnormality that may or may not be caused by trauma is spondylolysis. *Spondylolysis* is a break or defect in the pars interarticularis portion of the lamina (Fig. 5-13). It can be seen in about 5% of asymptomatic individuals. On oblique views the posterior elements form the figure of a Scottie dog, with the transverse process being the nose, the pedicle forming the eye, the inferior articular facet being the front leg, the superior articular facet representing the ear, and the pars interarticularis (which means the portion of the lamina that lies between the facets) equaling the dog's neck. If a spondylolysis is present, the pars interarticularis, or the neck of the dog, will have a defect or break. It often looks as if the Scottie dog has a collar around its neck. Although often difficult to visualize with MRI, spondylolysis should be easily seen on CT scans (see Chapter 11). The cause of a spondylolysis is said by some investigators to be congenital and by others to be post-traumatic. Many believe that this is a stress-related injury from infancy that develops when toddlers try to walk and repeatedly fall on their buttocks, sending stress to their lower lumbar spine. The significance of spondylolysis is just as controversial as its cause. More and more clinicians are coming to the viewpoint that a spondylolysis is an incidental finding with no clinical significance in most cases. Certainly some patients have pain related to a spondylolysis and get relief after surgical stabilization, but such cases are less common.

A   **B**

FIGURE 5-8 **Hangman's fracture.** *A,* A lateral film of a patient with a hangman's fracture shows an obvious example of the posterior elements of the C-2 vertebral body fractured and displaced inferiorly. *B,* The film of another patient shows a subtle fracture through the posterior elements of C-2 (*arrow*). A *line* drawn through the spinolaminar lines of the posterior elements shows the C-2 spinolaminar line to be offset in this example.

A

B

FIGURE 5-9 **Flexion teardrop fracture.** This patient suffered hyperflexion in a car accident and came to the emergency department with severe neurologic deficits. A lateral radiograph of the lower cervical spine shows wedging anteriorly of the C-7 vertebral body with some displacement of the posterior vertebral line of C-7 into the central canal. A small avulsion fracture off the anterior body is also noted.

FIGURE 5-10 **Unilateral locked facets.** The C6-7 disc space is abnormally widened, and the C-7 vertebral body is posteriorly located in relation to C-6. Also note the C-7 facets, which are dislocated and locked on the C-6 facets *(arrow).* When the facets are perched in this manner, the condition is termed locked facets, which in this example is unilateral.

FIGURE 5-11 **Unilateral locked facets.** *A,* The C6-7 disc space is slightly wider than normal, and the C-7 vertebral body is narrower in this view than the C-6 vertebral body, because of abnormal rotation. The facets of C-7 are not well identified, but in the tomogram *(B)* they are shown to be overriding and locked *(arrow).*

If a spondylolysis is bilateral and the vertebral body in the more cephalad position slips forward on the more caudal body, spondylolisthesis is said to be present (Fig. 5-14). *Spondylolisthesis* may or may not be symptomatic and by itself has no clinical significance. If severe, it can cause neuroforaminal stenosis and can impinge on the nerve roots in the central spinal canal. If it is symptomatic, it can be surgically stabilized.

A   **B**

FIGURE 5-12   **Seat belt fracture.** Hyperflexion at the waist can cause anterior wedging of the vertebral body in the lower thoracic or upper lumbar region as shown in A. By itself, this is somewhat innocuous; however, B shows a horizontal fracture through the right transverse process and pedicle *(arrow)* resulting from extreme traction during the flexion injury. When fracture of the posterior elements occurs, this injury is considered to be unstable and potentially debilitating. Any anterior wedging injury to a vertebral body should have the posterior elements of that level closely inspected for interpedicular space widening.

A   **B**

FIGURE 5-13   **Spondylolysis.** An oblique film of the lumbar spine (A) shows a defect in the neck of the Scottie dog at L-5 *(arrow)*, which is diagnostic of a spondylolysis. The drawing (B) shows the findings more clearly.

Anterior wedge compression fractures of the spine are commonly seen (Fig. 5-15), especially at the thoracolumbar junction, caused by an old injury; they are passed off by the radiologist, if they are mentioned at all, as incidental findings. The problem with this is you cannot tell from a plain film if the fracture is old or new, even if degenerative changes are present (which are often not related to the fracture). If acute and left unprotected, a wedge compression fracture can proceed

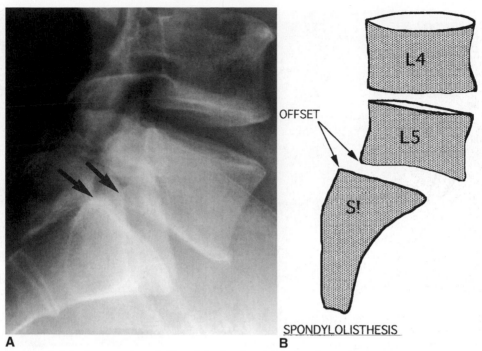

FIGURE 5-14 Spondylolisthesis. A lateral film of the lumbar spine *(A)* shows the L-5 vertebral body is slightly anteriorly offset on the S-1 body as noted by the posterior margins *(arrows)*. The drawing *(B)* shows the findings more clearly. Because the offset is less than 25% as measured by the length of the S-1 end-plate, it is termed a Grade 1 spondylolisthesis. A Grade 2 offset is more than 25% but less than 50% of the length of the S-1 end-plate.

to delayed further collapse with resulting severe neurologic deficits (Fig. 5-16). This is called Kümmell's disease, and it typically occurs 1 to 2 weeks after the initial trauma. I have seen over half a dozen lawsuits against radiologists who failed to mention minor anterior wedging of a vertebral body that went on to further collapse with associated paraplegia. All that needs to be mentioned is that a fracture is present that is of indeterminate age and requires clinical correlation. If the patient has pain in that location, a back brace needs to be worn until he or she is pain free. Old films can help to determine if it is an old fracture. If no pain is present on physical examination, it can be safely assumed to be an old fracture. It is not necessary to obtain a CT or MRI examination even if pain is present, because the treatment will be the same regardless of what the CT or MRI reveal. No spine surgeon will operate on a stable spine fracture without kyphosis or neurologic deficits, therefore the CT or MRI adds nothing but time and expense.

Patients who have fusion of their spine from ankylosing spondylitis, and, to a lesser extent, from diffuse idiopathic skeletal hyperostosis (see Chapter 6), are at a high risk for spinal fractures from even relatively minor trauma. Patients with ankylosing spondylitis typically have marked osteoporosis, which further magnifies their risk for fracture. A fused spine is more likely to fracture than a normal spine in a manner similar to a long glass pipette breaking more easily than a short one because it has a long lever arm. A small force at one end is greatly magnified farther down the lever arm. For that reason, a patient with ankylosing spondylitis should be treated as though a spinal fracture is present if they have back pain after trauma. CT and/or MRI are mandatory if plain films are negative (Fig. 5-17).

HAND AND WRIST

Several seemingly innocuous fractures in the hand require surgical fixation rather than just casting and, therefore, should be recognized by the radiologist as serious injuries. One such fracture is a fracture at the base of the thumb into the carpometacarpal joint, or a *Bennett's fracture* (Fig. 5-18). Because of the insertion of the strong thumb adductors at the base of the thumb, it is almost impossible to keep the metacarpal from sliding off its proper alignment. It almost always requires internal fixation. The radiologist occasionally has to remind a nonorthopedic practitioner of this, as well as closely examine the alignment of a Bennett's fracture in plaster that has not been internally fixed with pins.

A comminuted fracture of the base of the thumb that extends into the joint has been termed a *Rolando's fracture* (Fig. 5-19), and a fracture of the

FIGURE 5-15 Anterior wedge compression fracture.
Anterior compression of this lower thoracic spine vertebral body (*arrow*) is present, which may or may not be
acute. If the patient has pain in this area, it is most likely
acute and must be protected with a back brace until the
symptoms abate.

base of the thumb that does not involve the joint
has been called a pseudo-Bennett's fracture.

A *mallet finger* or *baseball finger* is an avulsion
injury at the base of the distal phalanx (Fig. 5-20)
where the extensor digitorum tendon inserts. With
the extensor tendon inoperative, the distal phalanx
flexes without opposition. If not properly treated,
this can result in a flexion deformity and inability
to extend the distal phalanx.

Another innocent-appearing fracture that often
requires internal fixation is an avulsion on the
ulnar aspect of the first metacarpophalangeal joint
(Fig. 5-21), which is where the ulnar collateral ligament of the thumb inserts. If the ulnar collateral
ligament is torn, the function of the thumb can be
impaired; therefore, this fracture can have a serious
result if not properly treated. This injury is called a
gamekeeper's thumb because of the propensity of
old English game wardens to acquire it from breaking rabbits' necks between their thumbs and fore-
fingers. A more current scenario is falling on a ski

A

B

FIGURE 5-16 Kümmell's disease. *A,* Minimal anterior
wedging of the L1 vertebral body is noted by comparing
the height of the anterior body versus the posterior
height. This patient had been in an auto accident and
complained of back pain. No treatment for his back was
given. *B,* After several weeks of continuing pain he presents with leg weakness that proceeded to paraplegia. A
spine film now shows progression of the vertebral body
collapse of L1. This almost certainly could have been
avoided with simple bracing of the spine after the initial
injury.

A   **B**

FIGURE 5-17 **Spine fracture in ankylosing spondylitis.** *A,* A lateral spine plain film after trauma shows fusion of the spine anteriorly, which was secondary to ankylosing spondylitis. Minimal anterior wedging of the L1 vertebral body is present that had been overlooked. *B,* Two weeks later, a CT scan of the spine was performed because of the sudden onset of paralysis. This axial image through L1 shows a fracture of the posterior elements that was undoubtedly present on the initial visit to the ER. Patients with ankylosing spondylitis need to be examined closely for any back pain after trauma and imaged with CT or MRI if any pain is present.

FIGURE 5-18 **Bennett's fracture.** A small corner fracture of the base of the thumb is noted that, at first glance, appears minor; however, it involves the articular surface of the base of the thumb *(arrow),* which makes this a serious injury that almost always requires internal fixation.

FIGURE 5-19 **Rolando's fracture.** A comminuted fracture of the base of the thumb that extends into the articular surface is a more serious type of Bennett's fracture and has been termed a Rolando's fracture.

FIGURE 5-20 **Mallet finger.** A small avulsion injury is noted at the base of the distal phalanx, which is where the extensor digitorum tendon inserts. This injury is termed a mallet finger or baseball finger. It is often caused by a baseball striking the distal phalanx, causing the avulsion. (Case courtesy Dr. Hideyo Minagi.)

pole and having the pole jam into the webbing between the thumb and index finger. Kayakers occasionally suffer a gamekeeper's thumb when their paddles hit a rock. This avulsion injury usually requires pinning to securely fix the ligament.

A fall on the outstretched arm can result in any number of wrist fractures and dislocations. One such serious injury is the *lunate/perilunate dislocation*. This dislocation occurs when the ligaments between the capitate and the lunate are disrupted,

FIGURE 5-21 **Gamekeeper's thumb.** A small avulsion injury on the ulnar aspect of the first metacarpophalangeal joint *(arrow)* is diagnostic of a gamekeeper's thumb. This is the insertion site for the ulnar collateral ligament and usually requires internal fixation.

FIGURE 5-22 **Normal lateral radiograph of the wrist.** The normal lateral view should show the lunate (L) seated in the distal radius and the capitate (C) in turn seated in the lunate. A line drawn through the radius should connect all three structures. Compare this radiograph with the drawing in Figure 5-23A.

Figure 5-23 Schematic depiction of normal lateral wrist (A), perilunate dislocation (B), and lunate dislocation (C). (The *dark shaded* bone is the lunate; the *cross-hatched filled* bone is the capitate. Ventral is to the left.)

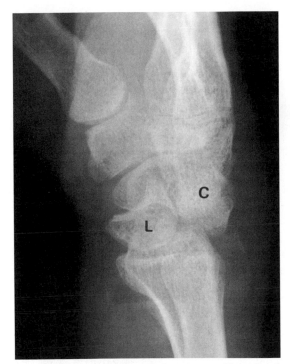

FIGURE 5-24 **Perilunate dislocation.** Although the lunate (L) is normal in relation to the distal radius, the capitate (C) and the remainder of the wrist are dorsally displaced in relation to the lunate. Compare this radiograph with the drawing in Figure 5-23B.

allowing the capitate to dislocate from the cup-shaped articulation of the lunate. This is best seen on the lateral view. Ordinarily, on the lateral view, the capitate should be seen seated in the cup-shaped

lunate (Figs. 5-22 and 5-23A). In a *dorsal perilunate dislocation* (occasionally the capitate dislocates volarly, but this is uncommon), the capitate and all of its surrounding bones, including the metacarpals, come to lie dorsal to a line drawn up through the radius and the lunate (Figs. 5-23B and 5-24). If the capitate then pushes the lunate volarly and tips it over, the line drawn up through the radius shows the lunate volarly displaced, and the line goes through the capitate. This has been termed a *lunate dislocation* (Figs. 5-23C and 5-25). The normal, perilunate, and lunate dislocations are shown schematically in Figure 5-23. Often it is difficult to tell whether the lunate or the capitate is displaced merely by drawing a line up the radius, because it can lie between the lunate and the capitate. In such cases, the designation of lunate or perilunate is difficult or even impossible. In reality, these are all perilunate-type dislocations, and additional trauma or manipulation of the wrist can cause the so-called lunate dislocation. It is certainly possible to turn a perilunate dislocation into a lunate dislocation merely by manipulating the wrist. Therefore, strict classification of these entities is not recommended by everyone. For many surgeons it is a moot point—they want rapid reduction of the capitate-lunate dislocation and don't really care which one happens to be more volarly or dorsally displaced. Failure to diagnose and treat this disorder can result in permanent impairment of the median nerve if it gets impinged by the lunate.

I strongly recommend that every radiologist get in the habit of looking at the alignment of the lunate and the capitate on every lateral wrist film. There's not a whole lot else to look for on the lateral view anyway. I see a missed perilunate dislocation every few years that usually ends up in litigation.

A lunate or perilunate dislocation can be diagnosed on an AP view of the wrist by noting a triangular or pie-shaped lunate (see Fig. 5-25B). Ordinarily, the lunate has a rhomboid shape on the AP view, with the upper and lower borders parallel.

Several fractures are known to be associated with a perilunate dislocation, the most common of which is a transscaphoid fracture. The capitate, radial styloid, and triquetrum also are known to frequently fracture when a perilunate dislocation occurs. Often, the fractures are identified and treated, whereas the dislocation is overlooked.

One of the most difficult wrist fractures to radiologically identify is a *fracture of the hook of the hamate.* A special view, the carpal tunnel view, should be obtained when trying to see the hook of the hamate. This view is obtained with the wrist (palm down) flat on a radiograph plate and the fin-

gers and palm pulled dorsally. The x-ray beam is angled about 45 degrees, parallel to the palm, so the carpal tunnel is in profile. The hook of the hamate is seen as a bony protuberance off the hamate on the ulnar aspect of the carpal tunnel. A fractured hook of the hamate can be seen with the carpal tunnel view (Fig. 5-26) but is often difficult to pick up. A CT scan will often show an obvious fracture that the plain film does not (Fig. 5-27) and should be considered in any possible carpal fracture when plain films are not diagnostic.

A fracture of the hook of the hamate most commonly occurs from a fall on the outstretched hand. A clinical setting that has gained attention in radiology and sports medicine circles is that of a professional athlete who participates in an activity in which the butt of a club, bat, or racket is held in the palm. Overswinging can result in the butt of the club levering off the hook of the hamate. This has been seen in professional baseball players, tennis players, and golfers. Why professionals? Amateurs usually are not strong enough to exert

A   **B**

FIGURE 5-25 **Lunate dislocation.** The lateral radiograph of the wrist *(A)* shows the lunate tipped off the distal radius, whereas the capitate seems to be normally aligned in relation to the radius yet is dislocated from the lunate. Compare this with the drawing in Figure 5-23C. The anteroposterior view *(B)* shows a pie-shaped lunate rather than a lunate with a more rhomboid shape. A pie-shaped lunate (L) is diagnostic of a perilunate or lunate dislocation.

FIGURE 5-26 **Fracture of the hook of the hamate.** The hook of the hamate is seen on a carpal tunnel view in this patient, as well as an area of sclerosis with a faint cortical break *(arrow)*. This represents a fracture at the base of the hook of the hamate.

FIGURE 5-27 **CT scan of a fractured hook of the hamate.** A CT scan through the wrist in this patient shows lucency in the left hook of the hamate *(arrow),* which represents a fracture. This could not be seen in the plain films, even in retrospect.

FIGURE 5-28 **Rotatory subluxation of the scaphoid.** An anteroposterior view of the wrist shows a gap or space between the scaphoid and the lunate *(arrow)*. This is abnormal and represents the "Terry-Thomas" sign, which means that the ligaments between the lunate and the scaphoid are ruptured. This is diagnostic of a rotatory subluxation of the scaphoid.

enough force to lever the hook off and, if they do, will usually terminate that activity, allowing healing. Professionals, however, continue their participation, which can lead to a nonunion of the fracture.

Another wrist injury that is seen after a fall onto the outstretched hand is *rotatory subluxation of the scaphoid.* This results from rupture of the scapholunate ligaments, which allows the scaphoid (navicular) to rotate dorsally. On an AP wrist radiograph, a space is seen between the scaphoid and the lunate (Fig. 5-28) when ordinarily they are closely opposed. This space has been called the "Terry-Thomas" sign, after a famous British actor with a gap between his two front teeth. The latest generation of radiologists is too young to have heard of Terry Thomas, therefore, I prefer to call it the "David Letterman" sign.

A *fracture of the scaphoid* is a potentially serious injury because of the high rate of avascular necrosis that occurs with this injury. When avascular necrosis occurs, usually surgical intervention and bone grafting are required to obtain healing. This fracture can be difficult to detect initially; therefore, whenever a fracture of the scaphoid is clinically suspect (trauma with pain over the snuffbox of the wrist), the wrist should be casted and repeat radiographs obtained in 1 week. Often the fracture is then visualized because of the disuse osteoporosis and hyperemia around the fracture site. Thus, in the acute setting, a negative film does not exclude a fractured scaphoid. Instead of casting the wrist and repeating the films in a week, many patients now get immediate MRI examinations to determine if a fracture is present (Fig. 5-29). This has been shown to be less expensive overall than having the patient cast and reexamined in a week.[4]

If avascular necrosis develops, it is the proximal fragment that undergoes aseptic necrosis, because the blood supply to the scaphoid begins distally and runs proximally. A fracture with disruption of the blood supply thus leaves the proximal pole without a vascular supply; hence, it dies. Avascular necrosis is diagnosed by noting increased density of the proximal pole of the scaphoid as compared with the remainder of the carpal bones (Fig. 5-30).

FIGURE 5-29 Scaphoid fracture. A coronal T1-weighted image of the wrist in a patient with snuffbox tenderness and a normal plain film shows a fracture of the midwaist of the scaphoid *(arrow)*.

Avascular necrosis can occur in other carpal bones, most commonly the lunate. This is called *Kienböck's malacia* and is most often caused by trauma, although some investigators claim it is idiopathic. The disease is diagnosed by noting increased density of the lunate bone, which may or

may not go on to collapse and fragment (Fig. 5-31). It often requires surgical bone grafting and occasionally removal or proximal carpal row fusion. Kienböck's malacia is said to have an increased incidence in patients who have shortening of the ulna in relation to the radius, called negative ulnar variance. Positive ulnar variance (the ulna is longer than the radius) is associated with an increased incidence of triangular fibrocartilage tears.

An avulsion fracture that is frequently seen is a *triquetral fracture*. The fracture is best seen on the lateral film, which shows a small chip of bone on the dorsum of the wrist (Fig. 5-32). This is virtually pathognomonic of avulsion off the triquetrum.

ARM

One of the most common fractures of the forearm is a fracture of the distal radius and ulna after a fall on the outstretched arm. This results in dorsal angulation of the distal forearm and wrist and is called a *Colles' fracture* (Fig. 5-33). When the fracture angulates volarly it is called a *Smith's fracture* (Fig. 5-34). A Smith's fracture is a much less common occurrence than a Colles' fracture. Sometimes the radius and ulna suffer a traumatic insult, and the force on the bones causes bending instead of a frank fracture. This has been termed *plastic bowing deformity of the forearm* (Fig. 5-35) and is often treated by breaking the bones (under

FIGURE 5-30 Avascular necrosis of the scaphoid. An anteroposterior view of the wrist shows a fracture through the waist of the scaphoid *(arrow)*. The proximal half of the scaphoid is slightly sclerotic in relation to the remainder of the carpal bones, which indicates avascular necrosis of the proximal half.

FIGURE 5-31 Kienböck's malacia. An anteroposterior view of the wrist reveals the lunate to be sclerotic and abnormal in shape. The lunate has collapsed because of aseptic necrosis. This is known as Kienböck's malacia. Note that the ulna is shorter than the radius—negative ulnar variance—which is said to be related to an increased incidence of Kienböck's malacia.

FIGURE 5-33 **Colles' fracture.** A fracture of the distal radius with dorsal angulation is noted, which has been termed a Colles' fracture (volar is to the left).

FIGURE 5-32 **Triquetral fracture and perilunate dislocation.** A perilunate or lunate dislocation is present (it is difficult to classify exactly which has occurred, because both the lunate and the capitate are out of their normal positions). Compare this radiograph with the drawing in Figure 5-23*A*. A small avulsion is seen on the dorsum of the wrist *(arrow)*, which is virtually diagnostic of an avulsion off the triquetrum. It is often associated with a lunate or perilunate dislocation.

anesthesia, of course) and resetting them. Left untreated, a plastic bowing deformity can result in reduced supination and pronation.

The forearm is a two-bone system that has some of the same properties as a bony ring. For example, a solid ring cannot break in only a single place; it must break in at least two points (try to break a pretzel—not a soft New York pretzel—in only one place). Likewise, the rings in the spine or pelvis always break in at least two places. In the forearm, a fracture of one bone should be accompanied by a fracture of the other. If the second fracture is not present, a dislocation of the nonfractured bone usually occurs. The most common example of this is a fracture of the ulna with a dislocation of the proximal radius (Fig. 5-36). This is called a *Monteggia's fracture.* (In previous editions of this book I termed this a "nightstick injury" from

FIGURE 5-34 **Smith's fracture.** A fracture of the distal radius with volar angulation such as this is called a Smith's fracture. This injury is much less common than the Colles' fracture shown in Figure 5-33 (volar is to the left).

FIGURE 5-35 **Plastic bowing deformity of the forearm.** These anteroposterior and lateral views of a child's forearm show the radius to be abnormally bowed. This condition has been termed a plastic bowing deformity of the forearm and occurs only in children.

police officers hitting someone with a nightstick [who hasn't had that happen!]—the person being hit instinctively raises an arm for protection and the nightstick falls on the ulna, fracturing it and dislocating the radial head. Lee Rogers called me and informed me that a nightstick fracture is a different entity than a Monteggia fracture. He's right, of course, but the mechanism I described is correct.) The dislocated radial head can be missed clinically and go on to aseptic necrosis with subsequent elbow dysfunction. Therefore, any time the ulna is fractured, the elbow must be examined to exclude a dislocation.

A fracture of the radius with dislocation of the distal ulna is called a *Galeazzi's fracture* (Fig. 5-37). This is much less common than a Monteggia's fracture, and because the deformity of the dislocated ulna is usually obvious, it is rarely missed clinically.

A helpful indicator of a fracture about the elbow is a displaced posterior fat pad. Ordinarily, the posterior fat pad is not visible on a lateral view of the

elbow because it is tucked away in the olecranon fossa of the distal humerus. When the joint becomes distended with blood secondary to a fracture, the posterior fat pad is displaced out of the olecranon fossa and is visible on the lateral view (Fig. 5-38). Therefore, in the setting of trauma, a visible posterior fat pad indicates a fracture. In an adult (epiphyses closed), the fracture site is almost always the radial head (see Fig. 5-38B). In a child (epiphyses open), it is usually indicative of a supracondylar fracture (Fig. 5-39). Often, the fracture itself is not visualized, and heroic steps are taken by clinicians and radiologists alike to demonstrate the fracture. These steps include oblique views, special radial head views, tomograms, and even CT scans and MRI. These are costly and unnecessary attempts to document pathology that will be treated identically regardless of whether it is radiographically recorded. So long as there is no obvious deformity or loose body, it does not matter if the fracture is definitely identi-

FIGURE 5-36 **Monteggia's fracture.** A blow to the forearm, such as with a police officer's nightstick, can result in a fracture of the ulna. Although the head of the radius appears normally placed on the anteroposterior view *(A)*, the lateral examination *(B)* reveals the head of the radius to be displaced. Failure to recognize this abnormality can result in death of the radial head with subsequent elbow dysfunction. This illustrates the importance of always obtaining two views of a bone in an injury.

fied in a patient with a post-traumatic painful elbow and a visible posterior fat pad.

Couldn't an infection cause a joint effusion and a displaced posterior fat pad? Of course, but the clinical setting would not be to rule out a fracture. In fact, any elbow effusion will cause a posterior fat pad to be visible.

The anterior fat pad also gets displaced with a joint effusion. Ordinarily, it is visible as a small triangle just anterior to the distal humeral diaphysis on a lateral film (Fig. 5-40). With an effusion it gets displaced superiorly and outward from the humerus and has been called a "sail" sign because it resembles a spinnaker sail (see Figs. 5-38 and 5-39). I have seen only one example of a displaced anterior fat pad without a visible posterior fat pad, and that was in a patient with a prior elbow fracture who probably scarred down the joint posteriorly,

preventing it from distending enough to push the fat pad out of the fossa. Therefore, I usually don't care what the anterior fat pad looks like and find it easier to concentrate on the presence or absence of the posterior fat pad. Keep things as simple as possible. Why be concerned over the appearance of two fat pads when one will do quite nicely?

Shoulder dislocations are generally easily diagnosed, both clinically and radiographically. The most common shoulder dislocation is the anterior dislocation. It is at least ten times more common than the posterior dislocation. For all practical purposes, these are the only two types of shoulder dislocations that warrant your concern.

An anterior dislocation occurs when the arm is forcibly externally rotated and abducted. This is commonly seen when football players "arm tackle," when kayakers "brace" with the paddle

A   **B**

FIGURE 5-37 **Galeazzi's fracture.** A fracture of the distal radius in this patient is seen on the anteroposterior view (*A*) without a definite fracture of the ulna. The lateral view (*B*) shows an obvious dislocation of the distal ulna, which would almost certainly not be missed clinically. This has been termed a Galeazzi's fracture and is much less common than a Monteggia's fracture.

above their heads and allow their arms to get too far posterior, when skiers plant their uphill pole and get it stuck, and as a result of similar athletic positions. Radiographically, the diagnosis is easily made on an AP shoulder film: the humeral head is seen to lie inferiorly and medial to the glenoid (Fig. 5-41). The humeral head often impacts against the inferior lip of the glenoid, causing an indentation on the posterosuperior portion of the humeral head called a *Hill-Sachs deformity*. A Hill-Sachs deformity is said to indicate a greater likelihood of recurrent dislocation, and some surgeons use it as an indicator to surgically intervene so as to prevent a recurrence. A bony irregularity or fragment off the inferior glenoid, which occurs from the same mechanism as does the Hill-Sachs deformity, is called a *Bankhart deformity*. This deformity is not nearly as common as the Hill-Sachs deformity.

A posterior dislocation can be a difficult diagnosis to make, both clinically and radiographically. An AP view may look normal, or nearly so. On the AP view of a normal shoulder, the humeral head should slightly overlap the glenoid (Fig. 5-42), forming a "crescent sign." In a patient with a posterior dislocation, this crescent of bony overlap is often absent and a small space is seen between the glenoid and the humeral head (Fig. 5-43).

The best way to unequivocally diagnose a dislocated shoulder is to obtain a trans-scapular view. An axillary view will show basically the same thing but requires the patient to move his arm and shoulder, which can be painful and can even redislocate the shoulder if it has already been reduced. The trans-scapular view is obtained by angling the x-ray beam across the shoulder in the same plane as the blade of the scapula. This gives an *en face* view of the glenoid, and the humeral head can easily be related to it as either normal, anterior (Fig. 5-44), or posterior (Fig. 5-45). Because of overlapping ribs and clavicles, the exact anatomy is often difficult to discern on the trans-scapular view. To find the glenoid, one has to find the coracoid, the spine of the acromion, and the blade of

A   **B**

FIGURE 5-38 **Displaced fat pads about the elbow.** On the lateral view of the elbow in this patient (*A*) the posterior fat pad is visible (*arrow*) and the anterior fat pad is elevated and anteriorly displaced (*curved arrow*). These findings indicate a fracture about the elbow, which in an adult should be in the radial head. An oblique view in this patient (*B*) shows the fracture of the radial head (*arrow*). Even without definitely seeing the fracture on the radiographs, it should be surmised to be present when the posterior fat pad is visualized in the setting of trauma. The elevated and displaced anterior fat pad has been termed a "sail" sign because it resembles a spinnaker sail.

FIGURE 5-39 **Displaced elbow fat pads.** A lateral view of the elbow in this patient shows a posterior fat pad (*arrow*) and a "sail" sign anteriorly (*curved arrow*). This is indicative of a fracture about the elbow, which in a child (the epiphyses are open) usually means a supracondylar fracture.

FIGURE 5-40 **Normal anterior fat pad of the elbow.** Note the lucency just anterior to the humerus of this normal elbow (*arrow*) and compare this with the "sail" sign of the anterior fat pads in Figures 5-38 and 5-39.

99

FIGURE 5-41 Anterior dislocation of the shoulder. An anteroposterior view of the right shoulder shows the humeral head to lie medial to the glenoid and inferior to the coracoid process (C). This is diagnostic of an anterior dislocation of the shoulder.

FIGURE 5-43 Posterior dislocation of the shoulder. Note that the humeral head in this patient is slightly displaced from the glenoid on the anteroposterior view. This is termed absence of the "crescent sign" and is often seen with a posterior dislocation. Compare this with Figure 5-42.

FIGURE 5-42 Normal anteroposterior view of the shoulder. Note on this example of a normal shoulder that the humeral head slightly overlaps the glenoid. This has been termed the "crescent sign."

the scapula. These three structures all lead to the glenoid and form a Y around it. All one has to do to find the center of the glenoid is to find two of those bony landmarks—usually the coracoid and the blade of the scapula. The humeral head can then be found and its position determined.

I was once involved in a court case where an emergency room (ER) doctor and a radiologist both missed a posterior dislocation in a patient who fell and had shoulder pain. The diagnosis was made 2 weeks later and the patient needed surgery—he was left with some permanent shoulder disability. The radiologist's lawyer argued that a community hospital radiologist should not be expected to diagnose such a rare disorder, even though the "University radiologist" (me) said it should be routinely identified. You certainly cannot expect to pass boards if you miss a posterior dislocation on your examination—this is bread and butter radiology.

An entity that can be mistaken for a dislocated shoulder is a traumatic hemarthrosis that displaces the humeral head inferolaterally on the AP film. Because the anterior dislocation displaces inferomedially it should not be confused with this. The

FIGURE 5-44 **Trans-scapular view of an anterior dislocation.** This trans-scapular view of the shoulder is obtained by aiming the x-ray beam parallel to the shoulder blade. The coracoid process (C) can be seen anteriorly, and the spine of the acromion (A) can be seen posteriorly. Both of these structures extend inwardly and meet at the glenoid (G). In this example, the humeral head is seen to lie outside of the glenoid in an anterior direction.

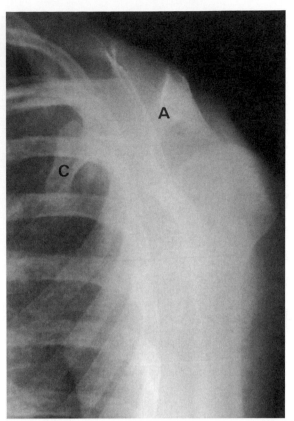

FIGURE 5-45 **Trans-scapular view of a posterior dislocation.** The trans-scapular view in this patient is more difficult to appreciate; however, the coracoid process (C) and the acromion (A) can still be identified, and the position of the glenoid (G) can be extrapolated. The humeral head is seen to lie posterior to where the glenoid lies.

posterior dislocation will easily be excluded by looking at a trans-scapular view. This is termed a pseudodislocation and is discussed more fully in Chapter 4.

If a fracture about the shoulder is suspected and the plain films are negative or equivocal, a CT scan should be performed. Any complex joint, such as the shoulder or hip, is best examined with CT scanning when the full extent of the fracture needs to be identified (Fig. 5-46).

PELVIS

Fractures of the pelvis, and especially those involving the acetabulum, can be difficult to evaluate completely with plain films alone. Because plain films often do not show free fragments and subtle fractures, CT scanning should be considered in almost all acetabular fractures (Fig. 5-47).

Sacral fractures are said to occur in half of the cases that have pelvic fractures, yet radiologists see a lot of pelvic fractures without seeing many sacral

FIGURE 5-46 **Fracture of the glenoid.** A CT scan of the shoulder in this patient who had a fracture identified on a plain film shows extension into the articular portion with a possible loose fragment (*arrow*). The plain film did not show the fracture extending into the joint.

A   **B**

FIGURE 5-47   **Dislocation of the hip.** *A,* An anteroposterior plain film of the left hip shows dislocation of the femoral head, which lies superior to the acetabulum. Fractures are easily identified on the CT scan *(B).* A cortical break through the articular surface of the posterior acetabulum, as well as the dislocation, is identified.

fractures. Why is this? Simple—we miss a lot of sacral fractures. They can be difficult to see on even the best of films because the sacrum is often hidden by bowel gas. In looking for sacral fractures, one should examine the arcuate lines of the sacrum bilaterally to see if they are intact. Fractures often interrupt these lines and, because of the side-to-side asymmetry, can be easily spotted (Fig. 5-48).

Sacral stress fractures occur commonly in patients who are osteoporotic or who have undergone radiation therapy. These present as patchy or linear sclerosis in the sacral ala that may or may not show cortical disruption (Fig. 5-49). They should be differentiated from metastatic disease because of their characteristic location, appearance, and history of prior radiation, and by the presence of a cortical break. These are often bilateral and then have a pathognomonic appearance on bone scan called a "Honda sign" (Fig. 5-50). They also have a characteristic MR appearance with geographic involvement of one or both sacral alae with low signal on T1-weighted imaging, which may or may not have high signal on T2-weighted imaging (Fig. 5-51).

Avulsion injuries affect the pelvis quite often and should be easily recognized by radiologists. On occasion, an avulsion can appear somewhat "aggressive," and if it is not diagnosed radiographically, a biopsy might be performed. This action can be calamitous, because avulsion injuries have been known to mimic malignant lesions histologi-

FIGURE 5-48   **Fracture of the sacrum.** An anteroposterior view of the sacrum in this patient shows normal arcuate lines on the left side of the sacrum that are interrupted on the right side *(arrows).* Interruption of these lines indicates a fracture through this portion of the sacrum.

cally, with a misdiagnosis leading to radical treatment (Fig. 5-52). Therefore, when an avulsion injury is a consideration, it becomes a "don't touch" lesion (see Chapter 4). Common sites for pelvic avulsion include the ischium, the superior and inferior anterior iliac spines (Fig. 5-53), and the iliac crest. Such injuries are fairly common in

A   **B**

FIGURE 5-49   **Stress fracture of the sacrum.** *A,* Faint sclerosis is noted in the left part of the sacrum as compared with the right in this patient describing pelvic pain. A radionuclide bone scan showed increased isotope uptake on the left half of the sacrum, and metastatic disease was postulated. A CT scan through this region *(B)* demonstrates a cortical disruption *(arrow)* indicative of a fracture. This is a characteristic plain film and CT scan appearance of a stress fracture of the sacrum.

FIGURE 5-50   **"Honda sign."** A radionuclide bone scan in a patient with bilateral sacral insufficiency (or stress) fractures shows increased uptake in the sacrum corresponding to an "H," which has been termed a "Honda sign." This finding is virtually pathognomonic for sacral stress fractures.

long jumpers, sprinters, hurdlers, gymnasts, and cheerleaders.

The symphysis pubis is another area in the pelvis that can demonstrate radiologic findings as a result of stress. In ultramarathoners, marathon cross-

FIGURE 5-51   **MRI of sacral insufficiency fracture.** A T1-weighted coronal MRI through the sacrum in the patient with the bone scan shown in Figure 5-50 reveals areas of low signal corresponding to the edema and reactive bone around the sacral stress fractures. Much of the area of low signal will get increased in signal on a T2-weighted sequence. Why get an MRI examination if the bone scan is pathognomonic? A good question. The MRI is certainly not necessary if the bone scan had been performed already, and the bone scan would not be needed if the MRI were the first study.

country skiers, and soccer players, the symphysis occasionally undergoes degenerative changes (Figs. 5-54 and 5-55). The hallmarks of degenerative disease (osteoarthritis) are sclerosis, joint space narrowing, and osteophytosis. In certain joints, however, erosions occur as a result of degenerative joint disease. These joints include the temporomandibular joint (TMJ), the acromioclavicular (AC)

A

B

FIGURE 5-52 **Avulsion off the ischium.** *A,* An antero-posterior view of the pelvis shows calcification extend-ing off the left ischium *(arrow)* in a patient reporting pain at this site. Note the irregular cortical surface, sug-gesting periostitis. *B,* The CT scan shows dense calcifi-cation adjacent to the ischium *(arrow).* These findings are characteristic for an ischial avulsion, and a biopsy should not be done.

FIGURE 5-53 **Avulsion from anterior inferior iliac spine.** A plain film of the pelvis shows a calcific density near the anterior inferior iliac spine *(arrow),* which is typical for an avulsion of the rectus femoris muscle.

joint, and the sacroiliac (SI) joint. These are easy to remember because they are the "letter joint"—the TMJ, the AC, and the SI. The symphysis pubis also behaves in this manner. Ordinarily when erosions are a feature of an articular process, osteoarthritis (degenerative joint disease) is not in the differen-tial diagnosis. It should be if the TMJ, the AC joint, the SI joint, or the symphysis is involved, however.

When the SI joints are involved with degenera-tive joint disease, the condition can closely resem-ble an HLA-B27 spondyloarthropathy (Fig. 5-56) and can lead to erroneous diagnosis and treatment. Large osteophytes can develop across the SI joints and mimic sclerosis (Fig. 5-57) or even a tumor (Fig. 5-58).

LEG

Overt fractures in the femur and lower leg are, for the most part, straightforward and deserve no

FIGURE 5-54 **Osteoarthritis of the symphysis pubis.** Sclerosis with erosion is noted at the symphysis in this ultramarathoner reporting severe pubic pain. This is char-acteristic of degenerative disease or osteoarthritis at this site in an overuse setting, such as in an ultramarathoner. Erosions are ordinarily not seen in degenerative disease except in certain joints, such as the symphysis pubis, the sacroiliac joints, and the acromioclavicular joints.

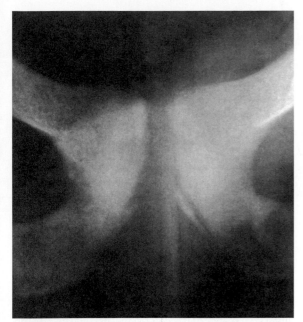

FIGURE 5-55 Osteoarthritis of the symphysis pubis. This is another example of sclerosis and erosive changes at the symphysis pubis in an ultramarathoner.

A

B

FIGURE 5-57 **Sacroiliac osteophytes.** An anteroposterior view of the pelvis (*A*) in this marathoner shows dense sclerosis over both sacroiliac joints. A CT scan through this area (*B*) demonstrates dense, bridging osteophytes characteristic of degenerative disease.

FIGURE 5-56 **Osteoarthritis of the sacroiliac joint.** Sclerosis and erosions (*arrow*) are seen in the left sacroiliac joint in this young, professional dancer. Although this finding has the appearance of an inflammatory arthritis, it also is seen in degenerative disease or osteoarthritis secondary to overuse.

FIGURE 5-58 **Sacroiliac osteophytosis.** A focal area of sclerosis is seen overlying the right sacroiliac (SI) joint (*arrows*) in this elderly patient. A metastatic process was a diagnostic consideration. This is characteristic, however, of an SI osteophyte seen in degenerative disease of the SI joints. (Case courtesy Dr. G. El-Khoury.)

special radiologic treatment for fear of missing subtle abnormalities. Stress fractures, however, need to be considered in anyone with hip or leg pain, because overlooking the diagnosis can lead to catastrophe. The most serious stress fracture—and fortunately one of the rarest—is the femoral neck stress fracture. It has been divided into three types by orthopedic surgeons: type 1—sclerosis without a fracture line evident (Fig. 5-59); type 2—a lucent fracture line without displacement (Fig. 5-60); type

FIGURE 5-59   **Femoral stress fracture.** An area of linear sclerosis (*arrows*) is seen at the base of the femoral neck in a neophyte runner with hip pain. This finding is diagnostic of a stress fracture of the femur. (Case courtesy Dr. David Simms.)

FIGURE 5-60   **Stress fracture of the femoral neck.** A linear lucency with surrounding sclerosis is seen in the femoral neck in this jogger with hip pain. This is a severe femoral neck stress fracture.

3—a displaced fracture is evident. The prognosis is best for a type 1 and worst for a type 3 fracture. Many surgeons believe that type 2 and type 3 fractures require internal fixation, whereas a type 1 fracture requires total bed rest for at least 3 to 4 weeks. Many type 1 fractures progress to complete fractures with displacement (type 3) with continued weight bearing; therefore, these are considered very serious lesions. If a femoral stress fracture is a clinical concern and plain films are normal, an MRI should be obtained.

Stress fractures also occur in the distal diaphysis of the femur and in the proximal, middle, and distal thirds of the tibia. All of these stress fractures need to be treated with the utmost caution, because complete fractures are not uncommon with continued stress (Figs. 5-61 and 5-62). Sclerosis in a weight-bearing bone that has a horizontal or oblique linear pattern should be considered a stress fracture until proved otherwise. Occasionally a stress fracture will appear somewhat aggressive, with aggressive periostitis and no definite linearity to the sclerosis (Fig. 5-63). If the fracture is mistaken for a tumor and a biopsy is performed, it can be confused with a malignancy, with subsequent radical therapy. Therefore, in such cases, a biopsy should not be done under any circumstances. If the clinical presentation is unusual for a stress fracture and the plain films are not diagnostic, take additional films 1 or 2 weeks later. Sometimes CT and MRI will better delineate the lesion. Stress fractures can be difficult to diagnose radiologically early on but should be straightforward after several weeks. A history of repetitive stress is not always obtained; therefore, the diagnosis should not depend solely on the history.

An unusual stress fracture is a fibular stress fracture (Fig. 5-64). The fibula is ordinarily not thought of as a weight-bearing bone, but in certain people it must serve as such.

One final stress fracture that deserves mention because it is frequently misdiagnosed clinically and overlooked radiographically is the calcaneal stress fracture (Fig. 5-65). It is often misdiagnosed clinically as a "heel spur" or plantar fasciitis and can be a subtle radiographic finding. MRI can be helpful in cases in which plain films are negative (Fig. 5-66).

Overt fractures in the lower extremity are uncommonly missed on radiographs; however, a few exceptions should be noted. Hip fractures in the elderly population can be difficult to detect (Fig. 5-67), and a high index of suspicion should be maintained. A negative plain film in an elderly patient with hip pain after trauma (even relatively mild trauma) does not exclude a femoral neck fracture. An immediate MRI should be obtained to exclude a fracture. MRI has proved to be useful in

A   **B**

FIGURE 5-61   **Stress fracture with completion.** *A,* A linear lucency is seen in the anterior cortex of the tibia in this runner, which is diagnostic for a stress fracture. *B,* This radiograph shows the result of continued exercise. The stress fracture went on to a complete fracture, which illustrates why any stress fracture of a long bone should be protected.

A   **B**

FIGURE 5-62   **Stress fracture with completion.** *A,* A faint linear sclerotic area *(arrow)* is seen, which is characteristic for a stress fracture of the proximal tibia. *B,* This radiograph shows the result of continued exercise in this patient: a complete fracture of the tibia and of the proximal fibula.

A   **B**

FIGURE 5-63 **Stress fracture of the tibia.** *A,* An irregular focus of sclerosis is seen in the posterior proximal tibia with adjacent periostitis. There was concern that this might represent a primary bone tumor, and the surgeons recommended a biopsy. An MRI scan was performed *(B),* however, showing a linear low-signal area running obliquely across the tibia, which is characteristic of a stress fracture. No significant soft tissue mass was found. The patient's recent history included an increase in his jogging, and a stress fracture was diagnosed on the basis of these images.

FIGURE 5-64 **Fibular stress fracture.** A linear band of sclerosis with adjacent periostitis *(arrow)* is seen in the distal fibula in this young female jogger. This is diagnostic for a stress fracture of the fibula.

FIGURE 5-65 **Calcaneal stress fracture.** A linear band of sclerosis is seen in the posterior calcaneus *(arrows),* which is diagnostic for a stress fracture of the calcaneus.

FIGURE 5-66   MRI of calcaneal stress fracture. *A*, A lateral plain film of the calcaneus in an elderly woman with heel pain and a history of lung carcinoma shows only osteoporosis. *B*, A radionuclide bone scan reveals diffuse increased uptake throughout the calcaneus. The question of whether to treat the calcaneus with radiation for metastatic lung carcinoma or to do a biopsy first was a dilemma. *C*, An MRI was obtained to get a better idea of where the met might be. This sagittal T1-weighted image shows a linear low-signal area (*arrow*) that is characteristic for a stress fracture. Obviously, no biopsy or radiation was necessary.

diagnosing hip fractures when plain films are negative (Fig. 5-68), and, even though expensive, it can actually reduce the overall costs by ensuring that no fractures are missed.

Another fracture that can be difficult to exclude on routine plain films is a tibial plateau fracture (Fig. 5-69). Many ERs routinely take a cross-table lateral view of the knee to look for a fat-fluid level in the suprapatellar recess. This finding indicates that a fracture has occurred and allowed fatty marrow to enter the joint; it has a high correlation with a tibial plateau fracture. In the appropriate clinical setting, tomograms, CT, or MRI may be necessary to make the diagnosis.

A

A

B

FIGURE 5-67 **Fracture of the hip.** *A,* An anteroposterior view of the hip was obtained in an elderly man after he had fallen. It was interpreted as normal, and the patient was released from the emergency department. Two weeks later the patient returned to the emergency department because he was unable to walk. Another radiograph was obtained *(B)*, and this shows a complete fracture through the femoral neck. In retrospect, the fracture can be faintly seen in *A* and should have been picked up initially. Fractures of the hip in the elderly can be difficult to see and should be diligently searched for with additional views when the clinical setting is appropriate.

B

FIGURE 5-68 **MRI of hip fracture.** *A,* A plain film of the hip in this elderly patient who has hip pain after a fall does not show a fracture. *B,* A T1-weighted MR shows linear low signal in the intertrochanteric region, which is typical for a hip fracture.

A

B

C

FIGURE 5-69 **Tibial plateau fracture.** *A,* An anteroposterior view of the knee shows no obvious abnormalities at first glance. However, a CT scan with reformations of the knee (*B*) demonstrates a plateau fracture of the lateral tibia. Note the rounded sclerosis, which, in retrospect, can be barely appreciated in *A. C,* A T1 coronal MRI shows a tibial plateau fracture that was barely discernible on plain films. MRI is an excellent imaging choice for subtle fractures. Tibial plateau fractures are probably the most commonly missed fractures about the knee.

A serious fracture in the foot that can be missed radiographically when little or no displacement occurs is the so-called Lisfranc's fracture (Fig. 5-70). It is named after a famous surgeon in Napoleon's army who would do forefoot amputations in patients with gangrenous toes after frostbite. The Lisfranc's fracture is a fracture–dislocation of the tarsometatarsals. If the dislocation is minimal, it can be easily overlooked. A key to normal alignment is that the medial border of the second metatarsal should always line up with the medial border of the second cuneiform and the medial border of the fourth metatarsal should line up with the medial border of the cuboid. If they do not, a Lisfranc's fracture–dislocation should be suspected. This fracture is seen most commonly as a result of catching the forefoot in something, such as a hole in the ground, or in a horseback rider falling and hanging by the forefoot

FIGURE 5-71   Boehler's angle in a normal calcaneus. This drawing shows the normal calcaneus with a line across the anterior process extending to the apex of the calcaneus, intersecting with a line from the posterior portion of the calcaneus to the apex. This is termed Boehler's angle, and when it becomes flattened or less than 20 degrees, a calcaneal fracture should be diagnosed.

FIGURE 5-70   Lisfranc's fracture. An anteroposterior view of the foot in this patient shows a space between the first and second metatarsals with the base of the second metatarsal displaced off the second cuneiform. This is indicative of a Lisfranc's fracture–dislocation.

FIGURE 5-72   Calcaneal fracture. Boehler's angle in this calcaneus is less than 20 degrees, which is indicative of a fracture of the calcaneus.

in the stirrups. It is not uncommonly seen as a neurotropic or Charcot's joint in diabetics. As with many fractures, MRI can be helpful in finding or excluding fractures when the clinical examination and the plain films are discordant.

A fracture of the calcaneus can be difficult to appreciate on routine radiographs. Boehler's angle is a normal anatomic landmark that should be looked for in every foot film when trauma has occurred (Fig. 5-71). If the angle is narrower than 20 degrees, a compression of the calcaneus is indicated, such as is seen with jumping injuries (Fig. 5-72). This fracture has been termed a "lover's fracture," for the propensity of lovers to jump out of windows when discovered in compromising surroundings by apparently larger or armed jealous suitors.

This fairly simplified overview of some commonly overlooked fractures and dislocations should in no way be interpreted as a substitute for the more complete texts listed in the references. For most residents and medical students it can serve as a starting

point, however, and perhaps stimulate reading in more depth on some of the topics.

REFERENCES

1. Rogers LF: Radiology of Skeletal Trauma, 3rd ed. New York, Churchill Livingstone, 2002.
2. Harris JH Jr, Harris WH: The Radiology of Emergency Medicine, 4th ed. Baltimore, Lippincott Williams & Wilkins, 2000.
3. Rockwood CA Jr, Green DP: Fractures in Adults, 5th ed. Philadelphia, Lippincott Williams and Wilkins, 2001.
4. Dorsay TA, Major NM, Helms CA: Cost-effectiveness of immediate MR imaging versus traditional follow-up for revealing radiographically occult scaphoid fractures. AJR Am J Roentgenol 2001;177(6):1257-1263.

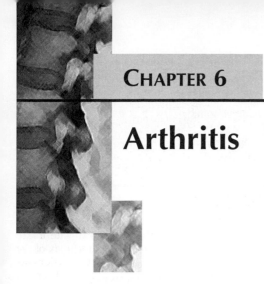

CHAPTER 6

Arthritis

The radiologic study of arthritis can be extremely difficult for the inexperienced because of the wide variety of patterns of disease, which produces a tremendous amount of overlap among the various diseases. What at first seems to be simple characterization of disease entities is found by the more experienced observer to be broad generalizations that may or may not fit into any one category of disease.

This chapter gives an overview of radiologic evaluation of arthritis with the caveat that it is, by necessity, a simplified version and in no way complete. If one is interested in greater detail or more accuracy, I would urge reading either Debbie Forrester's excellent monograph[1] on the subject or Anne Brower's superb book.[2] The definitive work on this subject is Don Resnick's six-volume tome,[3] but most can't read even the arthritis portion during a 4-year residency—it's best used as a reference.

The majority of arthritides are most easily examined and categorized by looking at their effect on the hands. Forrester[1] recommends a search pattern that she calls the ABCs, with the "A" indicating alignment, "B" standing for bone mineralization, "C" standing for cartilage and including a search for erosions, and the "S" standing for soft tissues. I would add to this search pattern by making it the ABCDs, with the "D" indicating distribution of the pathology. Although this is implied in Forrester's search pattern, I feel that it cannot be overemphasized.

In general, if the distribution of the arthropathy can be determined, the differential diagnosis becomes very short (Table 6-1). Although on paper this sounds quite nice, it can on occasion be difficult to accurately determine the distribution of the arthropathy. The distribution of the arthropathy is difficult to determine when it is not clearly distal or proximal but is more general, such as occurs with gout and sarcoid. It can also be difficult to accurately determine the distribution when

advanced disease is present, such as occurs with severe rheumatoid arthritis. With severe rheumatoid arthritis, the proximal nature of the pathology is not so apparent because of involvement with the metacarpophalangeal joints and even the phalangeal joints. In a similar manner, when psoriatic disease, Reiter's syndrome, or osteoarthritis is severely advanced, each can involve the more proximal portion of the hand and wrist, although this is unusual.

Side-to-side symmetry of the arthropathy is occasionally helpful in selecting a differential diagnosis (Table 6-2). Primary osteoarthritis and rheumatoid arthritis are classically described as bilaterally symmetric. Exceptions occur quite frequently, however, so that bilateral symmetry in these disorders is probably only on the order of 80 to 90%. Rheumatoid arthritis is a common offender of the bilateral symmetry rule, and one should not be surprised if rheumatoid arthritis is seen to be asymmetric in up to 20 to 25% of cases.

Involvement of joints other than the hand and wrist is not a common feature with most of the arthritides. In general, when a large joint such as the shoulder, hip, or knee is involved with arthritis, only a few entities need to be considered (Table 6-3). Although it must be emphasized that almost any arthritis can affect almost any joint, the diseases listed in Table 6-3 probably will account for 90% or more of the large joint arthropathies.

Involvement of certain joints often can give a clue as to the underlying disease process. For example, if the sacroiliac (SI) joints are involved, the differential diagnosis is as listed in Table 6-4. Again, almost any arthritis can affect any joint, but if the SI joint is involved, using Table 6-4 for the differential diagnosis will give a 95% or better chance of having the right answer.

Demineralization will occur around any joint that has pain, swelling, and hyperemia. Almost any

TABLE 6-1   Arthropathy Distribution in Hands and Wrists

Distal	Proximal
Psoriasis	Rheumatoid arthritis
Reiter's syndrome	Calcium pyrophosphate
Osteoarthritis	dihydrate crystal deposition disease

TABLE 6-2   Bilateral Symmetry of Arthropathy

Primary osteoarthritis
Rheumatoid arthritis

TABLE 6-3   Large Joint Involvement

Osteoarthritis (degenerative joint disease)	Ankylosing spondylitis
Rheumatoid arthritis	Pigmented villonodular synovitis
Calcium pyrophosphate dihydrate crystal deposition disease	Synovial osteochondromatosis
	Infection

TABLE 6-4   Sacroiliac Joint Involvement

Ankylosing spondylitis	Osteoarthritis (degenerative joint disease)
Inflammatory bowel disease	Infection
Psoriasis	Gout
Reiter's syndrome	Hyperparathyroidism

TABLE 6-5   Normal Mineralization

Osteoarthritis (degenerative joint disease)	Gout
Calcium pyrophosphate dihydrate crystal deposition disease	Pigmented villonodular synovitis
	Synovial osteochondromatosis

exceptions are exceedingly common. There are probably more missed diagnoses in the field of arthritis than in almost any other area of radiology. The remainder of this chapter gives a brief overview of arthritides with which most radiologists should be familiar. Rather than provide an in-depth description of each process—which can be obtained in any of the major radiology textbooks—I give salient discriminating points that might make it easier to differentiate one process from another.

OSTEOARTHRITIS

The most common arthritis seen by radiologists is osteoarthritis, or degenerative joint disease (DJD). It is believed to be caused by trauma—either overt or as an accumulation of microtrauma over the years. The hallmarks of DJD are joint space narrowing, sclerosis, and osteophytosis (Table 6-6; Fig. 6-1). If all three of these findings are not present on the radiograph, another diagnosis should be considered.

Joint space narrowing is the least specific finding of the three, yet it is virtually always present in DJD. Unfortunately, it is also seen in almost every other joint abnormality, so by itself it means little.

Sclerosis should be present in varying amounts in all cases of DJD unless severe osteoporosis is present. Osteoporosis causes the sclerosis to be diminished. For instance, in long-standing rheumatoid arthritis where the cartilage has been destroyed, DJD often occurs with little sclerosis. Osteophytosis also will be diminished in the setting of osteoporosis. Otherwise, sclerosis and osteophytosis should be prominent in DJD.

The only disorder that will cause osteophytes without sclerosis or joint space narrowing is diffuse idiopathic skeletal hyperostosis (DISH). This

of the arthritides can cause this to occur, yet there are a few entities that tend not to be associated with demineralization (Table 6-5). Normal mineralization in the presence of arthritis only indicates that there is no underlying hyperemia and probably no associated pain or at least long-standing pain at the time the radiograph was obtained. Normal mineralization often indicates an old, burned-out arthritis that was at one time painful and probably associated with demineralization. Nevertheless, when normal mineralization is noted around a joint that is abnormal, the entities in Table 6-5 should be strongly considered.

The above-mentioned differential diagnoses are to be considered generalizations and are, for the most part (except when mentioned), probably not more than 75 to 85% accurate. They are a nice starting point, however, for developing the differential diagnosis. I cannot overemphasize that the

TABLE 6-6   Hallmarks of Degenerative Joint Disease

Sclerosis
Osteophytes
Joint space narrowing

FIGURE 6-1 Degenerative joint disease of the shoulder. This former professional baseball pitcher with long-standing shoulder pain has joint space narrowing, subchondral sclerosis, and osteophytosis, which are hallmarks of degenerative joint disease (DJD).

FIGURE 6-2 Diffuse idiopathic skeletal hyperostosis. A lateral of the lumbar spine shows extensive osteophytosis without significant disc space narrowing or sclerosis. This is a classic picture for diffuse idiopathic skeletal hyperostosis (DISH).

common bone-forming disorder at first glance resembles DJD except there is no joint space (or disc space in the spine) narrowing and there is no sclerosis (Fig. 6-2). DISH is not believed to be caused by trauma or stress, as is DJD, and is not painful or disabling, as DJD can be. Millions of dollars per year are awarded to government employees on retirement for "disability" payments for supposed DJD acquired on their jobs, when in fact they have DISH and have been misdiagnosed. It is hoped that such errors will be rectified in the future as more radiologists become informed of the difference between DJD and DISH.

Osteoarthritis is divided into two types: primary and secondary. Secondary osteoarthritis is what radiologists refer to when speaking of DJD. It is, as mentioned, secondary to trauma of some sort. It can occur in any joint in the body but is particularly common in the knees, hips, and spine.

Primary osteoarthritis is a familial arthritis that affects middle-aged women almost exclusively and is seen only in the hands. It affects the distal interphalangeal (DIP) joints, the proximal interphalangeal (PIP) joints, and the base of the thumb in a bilaterally symmetric fashion (Fig. 6-3). If the arthritis is not bilaterally symmetric, the diagnosis of primary osteoarthritis should be questioned (Fig. 6-4).

A type of primary osteoarthritis that can be painful and debilitating is erosive osteoarthritis. It has the identical distribution as mentioned for primary osteoarthritis but is associated with severe osteoporosis of the hands and with erosions. It is somewhat uncommon, and radiologists generally see little of this disorder. Residents tend to mention erosive osteoarthritis in every example of joint erosions encountered whether it is in the hands, knees, hips, or wherever. This is totally inappropriate because erosive osteoarthritis only occurs in the hands, and there it has a characteristic distribution, which should make for an easy diagnosis.

There are a few exceptions to the classic triad of findings seen in DJD (sclerosis, narrowing, and osteophytes). Several joints also exhibit erosions as a manifestation of DJD. I call these joints the "letter joints" because they are all often called by their initials: the TMJ (temporomandibular joint), the AC (acromioclavicular) joint, and the SI joints; the symphysis pubis behaves similarly (Table 6-7). When erosions are seen in one of these joints, DJD must be considered, or inappropriate treatment can be expected (Fig. 6-5).

Another process that can occasionally be seen in DJD is a subchondral cyst or geode (taken from the geologic term used when a volcanic rock has a gas pocket that leaves a large cavity in the rock).

A   B

FIGURE 6-3 **Primary osteoarthritis.** A radiograph of the left (*A*) and right (*B*) hands in a patient with primary osteoarthritis shows classic findings of osteophytosis, joint space narrowing, and sclerosis at the distal interphalangeal joints, the proximal interphalangeal joints, and the base of the thumb. This was bilaterally symmetric in this patient, which is typical for primary osteoarthritis.

FIGURE 6-4 **Lack of bilateral symmetry in primary osteoarthritis.** This patient has classic radiographic findings of primary osteoarthritis in the left hand; however, the right hand shows only osteoporosis and soft tissue wasting without evidence of osteoarthritis. The reason for the lack of bilaterality is that this patient has long-standing right-sided paralysis, which has blocked the onset of the arthritic changes in the right hand.

TABLE 6-7	Joints That Exhibit Erosions with Osteoarthritis	
Temporomandibular (TMJ)	Acromioclavicular (AC)	
Sacroiliac (SI)	Symphysis pubis	

FIGURE 6-5 **Osteoarthritis of the SI joint.** A young woman, who is a professional dancer, described left-sided hip pain. This anteroposterior film of the pelvis demonstrated left SI joint sclerosis, joint irregularity, and erosions. A complete workup to rule out an HLA-B27 spondyloarthropathy was negative, and no laboratory or clinical evidence for infection was found. Her clinical history pointed to this process being completely occupation related, and an aspiration biopsy to rule out infection was therefore not performed. This is not an unusual appearance for DJD of the SI joints.

FIGURE 6-6 **Subchondral cyst or geode of the shoulder.** This patient has marked DJD of the shoulder with joint space narrowing, sclerosis, and osteophytosis. A large lytic process (*arrows*) seen in the humeral head is a subchondral cyst or geode, which often occurs in association with DJD. Because of the DJD in the shoulder, a biopsy to rule out a more sinister lesion in the humeral head should be avoided.

Geodes are cystic formations that occur around joints in a variety of disorders (Table 6-8). Presumably, one method by which they form is synovial fluid being forced into the subchondral bone, causing a cystic collection of joint fluid. They seldom cause problems by themselves but are often misdiagnosed as something more sinister (Fig. 6-6; see Chapter 4).

RHEUMATOID ARTHRITIS

Rheumatoid arthritis is a connective tissue disorder of unknown cause that can affect any synovial-lined joint in the body. The radiographic hallmarks are soft tissue swelling, osteoporosis, joint space narrowing, and marginal erosions (Table 6-9). In the hands, it is classically a proximal process that is bilaterally symmetrical (Fig. 6-7). There are so many exceptions to these rules, however, that I have come to regard them as no better than 80% accurate. Rheumatoid arthritis has a large variety of appearances and can often be difficult to diagnose with any degree of assurance from its radiographic appearance alone.

Rheumatoid arthritis in large joints is fairly characteristic in that it causes a lot of joint space narrowing and is associated with marked osteoporosis. Erosions may or may not be present and tend to be marginal—that is, away from the weight-bearing portion of the joint. In the hip the femoral head tends to migrate axially, whereas in osteoarthritis it tends to migrate superolaterally

TABLE 6-8	Diseases That Cause Subchondral Cysts (Geodes)	
Rheumatoid arthritis	Calcium pyrophosphate	
Degenerative joint disease	dihydrate crystal	
Avascular necrosis	deposition disease	

TABLE 6-9	Hallmarks of Rheumatoid Arthritis	
Proximal and bilaterally symmetric (hands)	Osteoporosis	
	Joint space narrowing	
Soft tissue swelling	Marginal erosions	

FIGURE 6-7   Rheumatoid arthritis. An erosive arthritis that primarily affects the carpal bones and the metacarpophalangeal joints is seen that has osteoporosis and soft tissue swelling (note the soft tissue over the ulnar styloid processes). It is a bilaterally symmetrical process in this patient, which is classic.

(Figs. 6-8 and 6-9). In the shoulder the humeral head tends to be "high-riding" (Fig. 6-10). Other things to think of when confronted with a high-riding shoulder are a torn rotator cuff and calcium pyrophosphate dihydrate crystal deposition disease (CPPD) (Table 6-10).

When rheumatoid arthritis is long-standing, it is not unusual for secondary DJD to superimpose itself on the findings one would expect with rheumatoid. This picture of DJD differs somewhat from that usually seen in that the sclerosis and osteophytes are considerably diminished in severity as compared with the joint space narrowing (Fig. 6-11).

HLA-B27 SPONDYLOARTHROPATHIES

A group of diseases that was formerly called "rheumatoid variants" is now known as the "seronegative HLA-B27 positive spondyloarthropathies."

TABLE 6-10   Diseases That Cause a High-riding Shoulder

Calcium pyrophosphate dihydrate crystal deposition disease	Rheumatoid arthritis
	Torn rotator cuff

FIGURE 6-8   Routes of migration of the femoral head. Osteoarthritis of the hip tends to cause superior (S) migration of the femoral head in relation to the acetabulum, whereas rheumatoid arthritis tends to cause axial (A) migration of the femoral head in relation to the acetabulum.

What was wrong with "rheumatoid variants"? It was short and concise. It has been replaced with a polysyllabic mouthful that is perhaps more descriptively correct, but so what? This is the problem with most academicians—make it sound more erudite and

FIGURE 6-9 **Rheumatoid arthritis of the hip.** Note the severe joint space narrowing in this patient with rheumatoid arthritis. The femoral head has migrated in an axial direction with fairly concentric joint space narrowing. Minimal secondary degenerative changes have occurred, as noted by the sclerosis in the superior portion of the joint; however, these have been diminished somewhat by the osteoporosis that usually accompanies rheumatoid arthritis.

FIGURE 6-10 **Rheumatoid arthritis in the shoulder.** An anteroposterior view of the shoulder in this patient with rheumatoid arthritis shows that the distance between the acromion and the humeral head is diminished (*arrows*). Ordinarily this space is about one fingerbreadth in width to allow the rotator cuff to move freely. This is a common finding in rheumatoid arthritis and in CPPD or with a torn rotator cuff.

maybe everyone will think we're smarter than we really are. They shouldn't be so insecure. I liked "rheumatoid variants."

These disorders are all linked to the HLA-B27 histocompatibility antigen. Included in this group of diseases are ankylosing spondylitis, inflammatory bowel disease, psoriatic arthritis, and Reiter's syndrome. They are characterized by bony ankylosis, proliferative new bone formation, and predominantly axial (spinal) involvement.

One of the more characteristic findings is that of syndesmophytes in the spine. A syndesmophyte is a paravertebral ossification that resembles an osteophyte except that it runs vertically, whereas an osteophyte has its orientation in a horizontal axis. Sometimes deciding whether a particular paravertebral ossification is an osteophyte or a syndesmophyte is difficult on the basis of its orientation alone (Fig. 6-12). Bridging osteophytes and large syndesmophytes can have a similar appearance, with both having an orientation halfway between vertical and horizontal. How should one evaluate those examples? Easy—ignore them. Look at the other vertebral bodies and use the ossifications on them to determine whether

you are dealing with osteophytes or syndesmophytes. If no other level is involved, you might just have to make the diagnosis on the basis of something else. In other words, sometimes you just will not be able to tell one from the other.

Syndesmophytes are classified as to whether they are marginal and symmetric or nonmarginal and asymmetric. A marginal syndesmophyte has its origin at the edge or margin of a vertebral body and extends to the margin of the adjacent vertebral body. Marginal syndesmophytes are invariably bilaterally symmetric as viewed on an anteroposterior (AP) spine film. Ankylosing spondylitis classically has marginal, symmetric syndesmophytes (Fig. 6-13). Inflammatory bowel disease has an identical appearance when the spine is involved.

Nonmarginal, asymmetric syndesmophytes are generally large and bulky. They emanate from the vertebral body away from the end-plate or margin and are unilateral or asymmetric as viewed on an AP spine film (Figs. 6-12 and 6-14). Psoriatic arthritis and Reiter's syndrome classically have this type of syndesmophyte.

Involvement of the SI joints is common in the HLA-B27 spondyloarthropathies. The patterns of involvement, like the patterns of involvement of the spine, are somewhat typical for each disorder. Ankylosing spondylitis and inflammatory bowel disease typically cause bilaterally symmetric SI

FIGURE 6-11 **Secondary degenerative disease in the knee in a patient with rheumatoid arthritis.** This patient has a history of long-standing rheumatoid arthritis. An anteroposterior view of the knee shows severe osteoporosis and joint space narrowing. Secondary DJD is occurring as evidenced by the sclerosis and osteophytosis; however, these findings are out of proportion to the severe joint space narrowing. When DJD narrows a joint to this extent, the osteophytosis and sclerosis are invariably much more pronounced.

joint disease that is initially erosive and progresses to sclerosis and fusion (Figs. 6-15 and 6-16). It is extremely unusual to have asymmetric or unilateral SI joint disease in these two disorders. Another entity that can have bilateral SI joint erosions is hyperparathyroidism. Subperiosteal resorption along the SI joints mimics erosive changes. This is more commonly seen in children.

Reiter's syndrome and psoriatic arthritis can exhibit unilateral or bilateral SI joint involvement. It is said that it is bilateral about 50% of the time. It is often asymmetric when it is bilateral, but exact symmetry can be difficult to assess on plain films. Therefore, when it is definitely bilateral and not clearly asymmetric, I consider the SI joints to be in the bilateral symmetric category. This means that if I have a case with bilateral, symmetric SI joint disease, it could be caused by any of the four HLA-B27 spondyloarthropathies. If I have a case with unilateral (or clearly asymmetric) SI joint involvement, I can confidently exclude ankylosing spondylitis and inflammatory bowel disease; I would consider

FIGURE 6-12 **Psoriasis with syndesmophytes.** The large paravertebral ossification on the left side of the T12-L1 disc space *(open arrow)* is difficult to differentiate between an osteophyte and a syndesmophyte. Either could have this appearance. However, the paravertebral ossification at the left L1-2 disc space *(solid arrow)* definitely has a vertical rather than a horizontal orientation, as does the faint ossification seen at the T11-12 disc space *(small arrow)*. These definitely represent syndesmophytes. Therefore, it makes sense to logically assume that the ossification at the T12-L1 disc space is almost certainly a syndesmophyte as well. This patient has large nonmarginal asymmetric syndesmophytes, which are typical of psoriatic arthritis or Reiter's syndrome. This patient indeed has psoriasis.

Reiter's syndrome and psoriatic disease. In this example, I would have to also consider infection and DJD (don't forget that DJD can cause erosions in the SI joints) (Figs. 6-5 and 6-17), and in older patients, gout should be considered. Computed tomography (CT) is helpful in examining the SI joints and is considered by many to be the diagnostic procedure of choice because of the unobstructed view of the entire joint (Fig. 6-18).

That is, in a nutshell, my approach to the SI joints (see Table 6-4). Other considerations in the

FIGURE 6-13 **Marginal, symmetric syndesmophytes in a patient with ankylosing spondylitis.** Bilateral marginal syndesmophytes are seen bridging the disc spaces throughout the lumbar spine in this patient. This is a "bamboo spine" and is classic for ankylosing spondylitis or inflammatory bowel disease.

FIGURE 6-14 **Syndesmophytes in psoriatic arthritis.** Large, bulky, nonmarginal asymmetric syndesmophytes *(arrows)* are seen in this patient with psoriatic arthritis.

differential are too uncommon for me to worry about for the most part, and you shouldn't either.

Large joint involvement with the HLA-B27 spondyloarthropathies is uncommon (except for ankylosing spondylitis) but occurs often enough to warrant some background. In general, the arthropathy will resemble rheumatoid arthritis with the typical features thereof (Fig. 6-19). The

FIGURE 6-15 **Ankylosing spondylitis.** Bilateral, symmetric SI joint sclerosis and erosions are seen in this patient with ankylosing spondylitis. Inflammatory bowel disease could have an identical appearance. Although this is classic for these two disorders, it would not be that unusual for psoriatic disease or Reiter's syndrome to have this appearance. Hyperparathyroidism can also have this appearance. It would be unlikely for infection or DJD to be bilateral in this fashion.

FIGURE 6-16 **Fusion of the SI joints in ankylosing spondylitis.** Bilateral complete fusion of the SI joints in this patient with ankylosing spondylitis makes the SI joints totally indistinguishable. Inflammatory bowel disease could have a similar appearance. I have not seen other disease processes affect the SI joints to this extent, with the exception of long-standing paralysis.

FIGURE 6-17 **Psoriasis with SI joint disease.** Unilateral SI sclerosis and erosions are seen in this patient with psoriasis. Ankylosing spondylitis and inflammatory bowel disease virtually never have this appearance.

FIGURE 6-19 **Ankylosing spondylitis with hip disease.** An anteroposterior view of the pelvis in this patient with ankylosing spondylitis shows bilateral complete fusion of the SI joints. Concentric left hip joint narrowing is present with axial migration of the femoral head. The hip changes would be typical findings in rheumatoid arthritis or, as in this example, ankylosing spondylitis. Note the secondary DJD changes in the hip as well.

hips are involved in up to 50% of the patients with ankylosing spondylitis.

Small joint involvement, specifically the hands and feet, is not commonly seen in ankylosing spondylitis and inflammatory bowel disease and tends to resemble rheumatoid arthritis. Psoriasis causes a distinctive arthropathy that is characterized by its distal predominance, proliferative erosions, soft tissue swelling, and periostitis. The erosions are different from the clean-cut, sharply marginated erosions seen in all other erosive arthritides in that they have fuzzy margins with wisps of periostitis emanating from them (Fig. 6-20A). The

severe forms are often associated with bony ankylosis across joints (see Fig. 6-20B) and mutilans deformities. A fairly common finding is a calcaneal heel spur that has fuzzy margins as opposed to the well-corticated heel spur seen in DJD or after trauma (Fig. 6-21).

A

FIGURE 6-20 **Psoriatic arthritis.** *A,* Cartilage loss at the proximal interphalangeal joints of the third, fourth, and fifth digits in this hand is apparent, with erosions noted most prominently in the fourth digit. These erosions are not sharply demarcated but are covered with fluffy new bone, which are termed proliferative erosions. Note also the periostitis along the shafts of each of the proximal phalanges.

FIGURE 6-18 **CT scan of the SI joints in psoriasis.** A CT scan through the SI joints in this patient with psoriasis shows unilateral SI joint sclerosis and erosions *(arrows)* typical for psoriasis or Reiter's syndrome.

(Continued)

B

FIGURE 6-20, cont'd *B,* Advanced psoriatic arthritis. Fusion or ankylosis is apparent across the proximal interphalangeal joints of the second through the fifth digits. Several of the distal interphalangeal joints are also ankylosed. Severe joint space narrowing at the metacarpophalangeal joints is noted. This distal arthritis is typical for psoriatic arthritis in advanced stages.

Reiter's syndrome causes changes that are identical in every respect with those of psoriasis with the exception that the hands are not as commonly involved (Fig. 6-22). Therefore, I recommend storing the findings for psoriasis and Reiter's syndrome on a single neuron and saving the other for a phone number or something else.

CRYSTAL-INDUCED ARTHRITIS

The crystal-induced arthritides include gout and pseudogout (CPPD). Ochronosis and a few other arcane crystal deposition diseases are so rare that they don't deserve mention except to say that you will probably never see an example outside of a textbook or teaching file.

Gout

Gout is a metabolic disorder that results in hyperuricemia and leads to monosodium urate crystals being deposited in various sites in the

FIGURE 6-21 **Reiter's syndrome.** A lateral view of a calcaneus in a patient with Reiter's syndrome shows poorly defined new bone on the inferior margin of the calcaneus with a calcaneal spur that is also poorly defined. This is typical of psoriatic arthritis or Reiter's syndrome as opposed to the well-formed calcaneal spur in DJD.

body, especially joint cartilage. The actual causes of the hyperuricemia are myriad, including inherited, and are not germane to this discussion.

The arthropathy caused by gout is very characteristic radiographically, yet it is not commonly seen. Why is that? Because it takes 4 to 6 years for gout to cause radiographically evident disease, and almost all patients are successfully treated long before the destructive arthropathy occurs.

The classic radiographic findings are well-defined erosions, often with sclerotic borders or overhanging edges; soft tissue nodules that calcify in the presence of renal failure; and a random distribution in the hands without marked osteoporosis (Fig. 6-23). I know of no other disorder that typically has erosions with sclerotic margins; therefore, this is a very specific finding for gout. It typically affects the metatarsophalangeal joint of the great toe (called podagra) (Fig. 6-24). In advanced stages it can be deforming (Fig. 6-25). Patients with gout often have chondrocalcinosis because they have an increased chance of having pseudogout (CPPD). Up to 40% of patients with gout concomitantly have CPPD.

It is worth repeating that patients must have clinically evident gout for years before changes will be apparent on a radiograph, and it is getting to be uncommon to find such a case. Also, even though erosions with overhanging edges can occur with

FIGURE 6-22 **Reiter's syndrome.** An anteroposterior view of the great toe in a patient with Reiter's syndrome shows fluffy periostitis in the erosions adjacent to the interphalangeal joint of the great toe. Marked soft tissue swelling is also present throughout the great toe. These changes are typical in appearance and location for Reiter's syndrome or psoriasis.

FIGURE 6-23 **Gout.** Sharply marginated erosions, some with a sclerotic margin, are noted throughout the carpus and proximal metacarpals. These erosions are classic in gout. Note the absence of marked demineralization.

gout, they can occur in other disorders as well and are by no means pathognomonic.

Pseudogout

CPPD crystal deposition disease causes much confusion among radiologists and other specialists. It is actually quite simple if you don't read all the conflicting literature. First, what do you call it? Is it pseudogout or CPPD? Who cares? Call it either, or both, or Fred. Many academicians say that it should be called pseudogout only when symptoms are present. Do we call lung cancer something else if the patient is asymptomatic? Of course not. For all practical purposes the terms pseudogout and CPPD are synonymous, and argument over the issue is academic B.S.

CPPD has a classic triad: pain, cartilage calcification, and joint destruction. The patient may have any combination of one or more of this triad at any one time. Each of these signs and symptoms will be dealt with individually in some detail, but note

that two of the three are radiographic findings. This disorder is best diagnosed radiographically.

The pain of CPPD is nonspecific. It can mimic that of gout (hence the term pseudogout), infection, or just about any arthritis. It typically is intermittent over many years until DJD occurs and becomes the main cause of pain.

Cartilage calcification, known as chondrocalcinosis, can occur in any joint but tends to affect a few select sites in the overwhelming majority of patients. These are the medial and lateral compartments of the knee (Fig. 6-26), the triangular fibrocartilage of the wrist (Fig. 6-27), and the symphysis pubis. Chondrocalcinosis in these areas is virtually diagnostic of CPPD. When CPPD crystals occur in the soft tissues, such as in the rotator cuff of the shoulder, a radiograph cannot differentiate between CPPD and calcium hydroxyapatite (CHA), which occurs in calcific tendinitis. Some refer to the deposition of CHA crystals in soft tissues as HAD—*hydroxy apatite deposition*. It is by far the most commonly seen source of soft tissue calcification. HAD does not occur in the joint cartilage except in extremely rare cases; therefore, all chondrocalcinosis can be considered CPPD. This, for some reason, is confounding to many people. Many established academicians have a hard time accepting that if chondrocalcinosis is present, CPPD crystals are the only possible culprit. Monosodium urate crystals in gout are not radiographically visible. CHA does not occur in cartilage. In fact, no other radiographically visible crystal in cartilage has been described. It couldn't

FIGURE 6-24 **Gout.** A sharply marginated erosion with an overhanging edge *(arrow)* is seen in the metatarsophalangeal joint in the great toe in this patient with gout. This appearance and location are classic for gout, whereas psoriasis and Reiter's syndrome usually involve the interphalangeal joint and do not have erosions that are this sharply marginated.

FIGURE 6-25 **Advanced gout.** Marked diffuse and focal soft tissue swelling is present throughout the hand and wrist in this patient with long-standing gout. Destructive, large, well-marginated erosions, some with overhanging edges, are noted near multiple joints. The focal areas of soft tissue swelling are called tophi, some of which are calcified. These calcify only with coexistent renal disease.

be simpler: chondrocalcinosis equals CPPD. So what's all the fuss about? Beats me.

The joint destruction or arthropathy of CPPD is virtually indistinguishable from that of DJD. In fact, it is DJD. It's caused by CPPD crystals eroding the cartilage. There are a few features of DJD caused by CPPD that will help to distinguish it from DJD caused by trauma or overuse. The main difference is one of location. CPPD has a proclivity for the upper extremity: the shoulder, the elbow (Fig. 6-28), the radiocarpal joint in the wrist (Fig. 6-29), and the MCP joints of the hand (see Fig. 6-27); it also tends to involve the patellofemoral joint of the knee in an isolated manner, that is, with no DJD seen in the medial or lateral compartments. These areas are not normally involved by DJD from wear and tear (such as the DIP joints of the hand, the hip, and the medial compartment of the knee). When DJD is seen in the joints that CPPD tends to involve, a search for chondrocalcinosis should be

FIGURE 6-26 **Chondrocalcinosis in the knee.** Cartilage calcification, known as chondrocalcinosis, is seen in the fibrocartilage *(arrow)* and in the hyaline articular cartilage in this patient with CPPD.

FIGURE 6-27 **Chondrocalcinosis in the wrist.** This patient with CPPD exhibits chondrocalcinosis in the triangular fibrocartilage of the wrist (*curved arrow*). A small amount of chondrocalcinosis is also seen in the second metacarpophalangeal joint (*small arrow*). Triangular fibrocartilage calcification is one of the more common locations for chondrocalcinosis to occur.

FIGURE 6-28 **CPPD arthropathy.** DJD of the elbow is seen in this patient with CPPD. Note the joint space narrowing with minimal sclerosis and the large osteophytes (*arrows*). Osteophytes of this nature are termed "drooping" osteophytes and are often seen in CPPD. The elbow is an unusual place for DJD to occur except in the setting of CPPD or trauma.

made. If necessary, a joint aspiration for CPPD crystals may be necessary to confirm the diagnosis.

Occasionally, the arthropathy of CPPD accelerates, and severe destruction occurs to such an extent that a neuropathic or Charcot's joint is mimicked on the radiograph (Fig. 6-30). This has been termed a pseudo-Charcot's joint. It is not a true Charcot's joint because of the presence of sensation.

Three diseases have a high degree of association with CPPD: primary hyperparathyroidism, gout, and hemochromatosis. This is not a differential diagnosis for chondrocalcinosis. These diseases tend to occur at the same time that CPPD occurs. If the patient has one of these three disorders, he or she is more likely to have CPPD than is a healthy person. There is probably not a good reason to perform a workup for every patient with chondrocalcinosis for one of the three associated diseases, because they are so uncommon and CPPD is extremely common. Several texts list many other disorders that are supposedly associated with CPPD, such as acromegaly, diabetes, Wilson's dis-

ease, and hypophosphatasia, but the recent work in this field does not support these findings.

COLLAGEN-VASCULAR DISEASES

Scleroderma, systemic lupus erythematosus (SLE), dermatomyositis, and mixed connective tissue disease are all grouped together as collagen-vascular diseases. The striking abnormalities in the hands in each of these disorders are osteoporosis and soft tissue wasting. SLE characteristically has severe ulnar deviation of the phalanges (Fig. 6-31). Erosions are generally not present in these diseases. Soft tissue calcifications are typically present in scleroderma (Fig. 6-32) and dermatomyositis. Mixed connective tissue disease is an overlap of scleroderma, SLE, polymyositis, and rheumatoid arthritis. Obviously, it has a myriad of radiographic findings.

FIGURE 6-29 **CPPD arthropathy.** Marked DJD at the radiocarpal joint is seen in this patient with CPPD. Severe joint space narrowing and sclerosis with large subchondral cysts or geodes are hallmarks of DJD. This is an unusual location for DJD except in the setting of CPPD.

SARCOID

Sarcoidosis causes deposition of granulation tissue in the body, primarily in the lungs but also in the bones. In the skeletal system it has a predilection for the hands, where it causes lytic destructive lesions in the cortex. These often have a lacelike appearance (Fig. 6-33). Sarcoid also can affect the joints in the hand, causing DJD-like changes.

HEMOCHROMATOSIS

About 20 to 50% of patients with hemochromatosis have a characteristic arthropathy in the hands that should suggest the diagnosis. Hemochromatosis is a disease of excess iron that gets deposited in tissues throughout the body, leading to fibrosis and eventual organ failure. The characteristic arthropathy classically involves the second through fourth metacarpophalangeal

A   **B**

FIGURE 6-30 **Pseudo-Charcot's joint in CPPD.** This patient with CPPD shows severe joint destruction in the carpus primarily at the radiocarpal joint. Large subchondral cysts or geodes are noted (*A*). Heterotopic new bone or joint debris is also seen (*arrow*). *B*, Dislocation of the radiocarpal joint is seen, with the entire carpus lying volarly in relation to the radius. The findings of severe joint destruction, heterotopic new bone, and dislocation are classic for a Charcot's joint. This patient, however, had sensation in this joint; therefore, it is not a true Charcot's or neuropathic joint but a pseudo-Charcot's joint, which is occasionally seen in CPPD.

joints. The radiographic changes are essentially those of DJD (joint space narrowing, sclerosis, and osteophytes) (Fig. 6-34). Up to 50% of patients with hemochromatosis also have CPPD; therefore, when looking at the hands, a search should be made for triangular fibrocartilage chondrocalcinosis. Another finding that is often seen in hemochromatosis is called "squaring" of the metacarpal heads. They appear enlarged and blocklike as a result of the large osteophytes commonly seen in this disorder. In fact, the osteophytes are often called "drooping" because of the unusual way they hang off the joint margin.

NEUROPATHIC OR CHARCOT'S JOINT

The radiographic findings for a Charcot's joint are characteristic and almost pathognomonic. A classic triad has been described that consists of joint destruction, dislocation, and heterotopic new bone (Fig. 6-35). Multiple other findings have been described that do not seem to be as useful as the classic triad.

Joint destruction is seen in every arthritis form encountered and, therefore, seems very nonspecific; however, nothing causes as severe destruction in a joint as a Charcot's joint. Early in the develop-

ment of a Charcot's joint the joint destruction may merely appear to be joint space narrowing. It is extremely difficult to make the diagnosis this early. In the spine, instead of joint space destruction, there is disc space destruction (Fig. 6-36).

Dislocation, like joint destruction, can be present in varying degrees. Early on the joint may have subluxation instead of dislocation.

Heterotopic new bone has also been termed "debris" and consists of soft tissue calcification or clumps of ossification adjacent to the joint. It, too, can be present in varying amounts.

The most commonly seen Charcot's joint currently is in the foot of a patient with diabetes. It typically affects the first and second tarsometatarsal joints in a fashion termed a Lisfranc's fracture (Fig. 6-37). Lisfranc was Napoleon's surgeon, and he gained fame for saving the lives of soldiers with gangrenous toes from frostbite by doing a forefoot amputation at the tarsometatarsal junction.

Tabes dorsalis from syphilis is seldom seen today. I have only encountered one case of a Charcot's joint in syphilis in the last 25 years, and I've been around some pretty raunchy residents. More commonly seen is a Charcot's joint in a patient with paralysis who continues to use the affected limb for support.

FIGURE 6-31 **Systemic lupus erythematosus (SLE).** Marked soft tissue wasting, as noted by the concavity in the hypothenar eminence, occurs with ulnar deviation of the phalanges and is seen primarily in the right hand in this patient. These are hallmarks of SLE.

FIGURE 6-32   **Scleroderma.** Diffuse subcutaneous soft tissue calcification is seen throughout the hands and wrist in this patient with scleroderma. Soft tissue wasting and osteoporosis are also present, and bone loss in multiple distal phalanges secondary to the vascular abnormalities often present in this disease.

The shoulder can become a Charcot's joint in patients with syringomyelia, which has a so-called "atrophic Charcot" appearance. This refers to its tendency to have no debris or heterotopic new bone, and the proximal humerus has a tapered appearance likened to a licked candy stick.

A pseudo-Charcot's joint from CPPD (see Fig. 6-30) is encountered almost as commonly as a true Charcot joint from any other cause with the exception of the Lisfranc type seen in patients with diabetes.

HEMOPHILIA, JUVENILE RHEUMATOID ARTHRITIS, AND PARALYSIS

Why would two clinically disparate entities like juvenile rheumatoid arthritis (JRA) and hemophilia be covered in the same section? Because this is a radiology textbook, and these conditions are radiographically indistinguishable. As with several other processes covered in this book, you may as well store these two on a single neuron and save the other neuron for something important.

The classic findings for JRA and hemophilia are overgrowth of the ends of the bones (epiphyseal enlargement) associated with gracile diaphyses (Fig. 6-38). Joint destruction may or may not be present (Figs. 6-39 and 6-40). A finding that is purported to be classic for JRA and hemophilia is widening of the intercondylar notch of the knee. I find this sign variable and difficult to use. I have never seen it present when the other classic signs were not also present and obvious.

Another process that can mimic the findings in JRA and hemophilia is a joint that has undergone disuse from paralysis (Fig. 6-41). It has always been said that the reason the epiphyses are overgrown in JRA and hemophilia is because of the hyperemia; however, a lot of other things cause hyperemia without affecting the size of the epiphyses. The thing that JRA, hemophilia, and paralysis have in common is disuse. I believe that this is what causes the overgrowth of the ends of the bones seen in all three disorders.

SYNOVIAL OSTEOCHONDROMATOSIS

Synovial osteochondromatosis, a relatively common disorder, is caused by a metaplasia of the synovium, resulting in the deposition of foci of

FIGURE 6-34   **Hemochromatosis.** An anteroposterior view of the hand in this patient with hemochromatosis shows severe joint space narrowing throughout the hand, which is most marked at the metacarpophalangeal joints. Associated sclerosis at the metacarpopha-langeal joints with large osteophytes seen off the metacarpal heads suggests DJD. These are unusual joints for DJD to occur in, yet this is the classic appearance of hemochromatosis. No chondrocalcinosis is seen in the triangular cartilage in this patient; however, a small amount of chondrocalcinosis can be seen at the second metacarpophalangeal joint *(arrow).* About 50% of patients with hemochromatosis also have CPPD.

FIGURE 6-33   **Sarcoid.** An anteroposterior view of the hand in this patient with sarcoid demonstrates classic changes of bony involvement with this granulomatous process. Note the lacelike pattern of destruction seen most prominently in the proximal phalanges and the dis-tal third phalanx. Soft tissue swelling and some areas of severe bony dissolution are also noted, which occur in more advanced patterns of sarcoid. These changes are typically limited to the hands but can rarely occur in other parts of the skeleton.

cartilage in the joint. It is most commonly seen in the knee, hip, and elbow. Most of the time these cartilaginous deposits calcify and are readily seen on a radiograph (Figs. 6-42 and 6-43). In up to 30% of cases the cartilaginous deposits do not cal-cify. In these cases, all that is seen on the ra-diograph is a joint effusion unless erosions or joint destruction occur (Fig. 6-44).

The calcifications begin in the synovium and then tend to shed into the joint, where they can cause symptoms of free fragments or "joint mice." They then embed into the synovium and tend not to be free in the joint after a while. If the loose bodies are all of the same size, it is termed "primary" synovial osteochondromatosis. It is usually necessary to perform a complete synovec-tomy to relieve the symptoms. If the loose bodies are of different sizes, it is termed "secondary"

synovial osteochondromatosis. This indicates it is secondary to underlying DJD in which small bits of cartilage are shed into the joint and grow as they are nourished by the synovial fluid. Because the shedding of the joint fragments occurs at varying times, the loose bodies are of different sizes. The differentiation of primary versus sec-ondary synovial osteochondromatosis is impor-tant as the primary type requires a synovectomy, whereas the secondary type requires removal of the loose bodies and treatment of the DJD, but no synovectomy.

An uncommon presentation of synovial osteo-chondromatosis is tumefactive synovial osteochon-dromatosis. This occurs when the loose bodies are so tightly packed in a joint that it appears on MRI examination to be a solid tumor (see discussion and figures in Chapter 3).

FIGURE 6-35 **Charcot's joint.** An anteroposterior view of the knee in this patient with tabes dorsalis shows the classic changes of a neuropathic or Charcot's joint. Note the severe joint destruction, the subluxation, and the heterotopic new bone *(arrow)*.

FIGURE 6-36 **Charcot's spine.** An anteroposterior view of the spine in this paraplegic shows severe destruction of the L2 and L3 vertebral bodies and the intervening disc space, heterotopic new bone *(arrow)*, and malalignment or dislocation.

PIGMENTED VILLONODULAR SYNOVITIS

Pigmented villonodular synovitis (PVNS) is a chronic, inflammatory process of the synovium that causes synovial proliferation. A swollen joint with lobular masses of synovium occurs, which causes pain and joint destruction (Fig. 6-45). It seldom, if ever, calcifies. It has been termed giant cell tumor of tendon sheath and tendon sheath xanthoma when it occurs in a tendon sheath, which is not unusual. PVNS looks radiographically identical to noncalcified synovial osteochondromatosis, yet it is much less common. Therefore, whenever PVNS is a consideration, mention synovial osteochondromatosis (noncalcified). MRI examination of a joint with PVNS shows a pathognomonic appearance of low-signal hemosiderin deposits lining the synovium (Fig. 6-46).

SUDECK'S ATROPHY

Also known as shoulder-hand syndrome and reflex sympathetic dystrophy, Sudeck's atrophy is a poorly understood joint affliction that typically occurs after minor trauma to an extremity, resulting in pain, swelling, and dysfunction. Severe osteoporosis and swelling are seen radiographically (Fig. 6-47). The disorder typically affects the distal part of an extremity, such as a hand or foot, yet intermediate joints, such as the knee and hip, are thought by some to occasionally be involved. The pain usually subsides, but the osteoporosis may persist. The swelling, with time, will subside, and the skin may become atrophic. It is important for the radiologist to recognize the aggressive osteoporosis in this disorder so the treating physician can begin aggressive physical therapy.

JOINT EFFUSIONS

Radiology residents often go to great extremes to determine whether a joint—be it a knee, hip, shoulder, elbow, or whatever—has an effusion. There are some good signs of joint effusions (which I will review), and there are some that are used that are invalid. The thing that amazes me is

FIGURE 6-37 **Lisfranc Charcot's joint.** Dislocation of the second and third metatarsals together with joint destruction and large amounts of heterotopic new bone are present in the foot of this patient with diabetes. These findings are classic for a Charcot's joint that has been termed a Lisfranc's fracture–dislocation. It is most commonly seen secondary to trauma rather than as a Charcot's joint but currently is the most common neuropathic joint seen.

all the attention it gets, because when all is said and done, in most cases, it doesn't make any difference whatsoever. With the exception of the elbow (see Chapter 5), and possibly the hip, treatment is never predicated on the radiographic finding of a joint effusion.

Most joint effusions are clinically obvious and do not require radiographic validation. As mentioned earlier, the elbow is an exception. In the setting of trauma to the elbow, an effusion indicates a fracture. The radiographic signs of an elbow effusion are generally clearly seen and have proved to be valid. Clinical determination of an elbow effusion can be difficult; therefore, the radiologist can be helpful in this area.

Clinical determination of a hip effusion is also difficult. The presence of a hip effusion can be valuable in certain clinical settings. For instance, in a patient with pain in the hip and an effusion, the joint should be aspirated to rule out an infec-

FIGURE 6-38 **Juvenile rheumatoid arthritis (JRA).** A lateral view of the knee in this patient with JRA shows the classic findings of overgrowth of the ends of the bones and associated gracile diaphyses. These changes can also be seen in patients with hemophilia or paralysis.

tion. If only pain were present, an aspiration would probably not be performed. The radiology literature mentions displacement of the fat stripes about the hip as being an indicator for an effusion, but this has been proved to be fallacious. The only fat pad around the hip that gets displaced with an effusion is the obturator internus, and it is seldom seen. The remainder of the fat pads is far removed from the joint capsule and is not directly influenced by the joint.

A radiographic sign in the hip that does work for indicating an effusion is called the teardrop sign. Leonard Swischuk first brought this sign to my attention by its application in pediatric patients. I have used it in adults as well with good results. The teardrop is an anatomic landmark at the medial aspect of the hip joint (Fig. 6-48) that is made up of several bony structures bounding the acetabulum medially. The teardrop measurement is the distance from the most medial part of the femoral head to the most medial extent of the acetabulum (which is the teardrop). This measurement—inappropriately called the teardrop measurement—should be equal in both hips. An effusion will push the femoral head laterally and give the affected side a wider teardrop distance (Fig. 6-49). The teardrop distance is a valid indicator of an effusion in children. It is valid in adults only when no long-standing joint abnormality,

FIGURE 6-39 **Hemophilia.** An anteroposterior view of the ankle in this patient with hemophilia shows subtle changes of overgrowth of the distal tibia and fibula as compared with the diameter of the diaphyses. Some joint destruction of the tibiotalar joint is also noted.

FIGURE 6-40 **Hemophilia.** An anterior view of the elbow in this patient with hemophilia shows overgrowth of the ends of the bones, in particular the head of the radius, and marked joint destruction. JRA could certainly cause an appearance such as this.

FIGURE 6-41 **Muscular dystrophy.** This patient with muscular dystrophy has changes similar to those of JRA and hemophilia, which consist of overgrowth of the ends of the bones and a tibiotalar slant. This appearance is frequently found in patients with paralysis.

such as DJD or an old fracture, is present. A difference in the teardrop distance from one hip to the other of as little as 1 mm is significant in the appropriate clinical setting. It would be better to aspirate a few normal hips rather than risk missing a hip infection that might destroy the hip if diagnosed late.

The radiographic sign for a knee effusion that seems to be the most reliable is the measurement of the distance between the suprapatellar fat pad and the anterior femoral fat pad (Fig. 6-50). A distance between these two fat pads of more than 10 mm is definite evidence for an effusion. A distance of less than 5 mm is normal. A distance of 5 to 10 mm is no man's land. I usually call it an effusion if the distance is greater than 5 mm, realizing that I'm probably overcalling a few. I am also aware that it doesn't make any difference if there is an effusion in the knee or not—the patient gets treated the same regardless. If it were vital to the patient, you could aspirate the joint or perform an MRI study to

FIGURE 6-42 Synovial osteochondromatosis. An anteroposterior view of the hip in this patient with left hip pain shows multiple calcified loose bodies in the hip joint. The loose bodies are all of a similar size; therefore, this is diagnostic of primary synovial osteochondromatosis.

FIGURE 6-44 Synovial osteochondromatosis without calcification. An anteroposterior view of the hip in this patient shows the femoral neck to be virtually whittled down, with the femoral head undercut, giving an apple core appearance. This has occurred from the pressure erosion of multiple nonossified loose bodies in the joint. This is nonossified synovial osteochondromatosis, which is probably more properly termed synovial chondromatosis. It usually does not cause this degree of bony erosion and is indistinguishable from pigmented villonodular synovitis.

FIGURE 6-43 Synovial osteochondromatosis. Multiple calcified loose bodies are seen in the suprapatellar space of the knee in this patient. The loose bodies are of different sizes; therefore, this is diagnostic of secondary synovial osteochondromatosis.

FIGURE 6-45 Pigmented villonodular synovitis (PVNS). An anteroposterior view of the hip in this patient shows joint space destruction and bony erosions throughout the femoral head and neck. PVNS or synovial chondromatosis (nonossified) could have this appearance.

A

B

FIGURE 6-46 **Pigmented villonodular synovitis (PVNS).** Sagittal T1-weighted *(A)* and fast spin echo (FSE) T2-weighted *(B)* images of an ankle with PVNS show a soft tissue mass emanating from the ankle joint, which is low signal on both sequences, and has very low-signal hemosiderin lining parts of the synovium, which is characteristic for PVNS.

find out. I should emphasize that we never do an MR examination just to see if there is fluid in the joint.

Shoulder effusions are difficult to detect unless they are massive enough to displace the humeral head inferiorly, as with a fracture and hemarthrosis (see Chapter 5). Fortunately, as with most other joints, treatment is not based on the presence or absence of an effusion, therefore it hardly matters.

FIGURE 6-47 **Sudeck's atrophy.** Diffuse soft tissue swelling and marked osteoporosis that is so aggressive it has a spotty or permeative appearance around the joints is noted in this patient with severe hand pain and dysfunction after minor trauma. This is characteristic of Sudeck's atrophy.

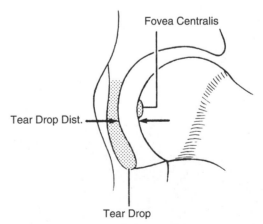

FIGURE 6-48 **Drawing of the teardrop measurement.** The teardrop measurement is the distance from the most medial aspect of the femoral head to the nearest portion of the adjacent acetabulum *(arrows)*. Widening of this distance as compared with the opposite hip is indicative of a joint effusion.

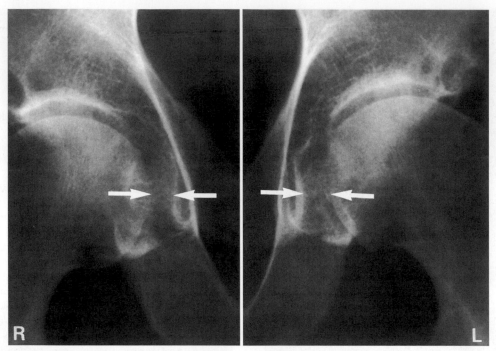

FIGURE 6-49 **Widened teardrop.** The teardrop distance in this patient on the left side (*arrows*) is slightly wider than that on the right side (*arrows*), which is indicative of a hip joint effusion. This patient had a hip joint infection on the left side.

FIGURE 6-50 **Knee joint effusion.** This patient has a fractured patella with a large joint effusion. The suprapatellar pouch is grossly distended, with the distance between the suprapatellar fat pad and the anterior femoral fat pad measuring more than 1.0 cm (*arrows*).

The same is true in the ankle, wrist, and smaller joints.

AVASCULAR NECROSIS

Avascular necrosis (AVN), or aseptic necrosis, can occur around almost any joint for a host of reasons, including steroid use, trauma, various underlying disease states, and even idiopathically. It is often seen in patients who have received renal transplants.

The hallmark of AVN is increased bone density at an otherwise normal joint. Increased density at a joint usually indicates DJD; however, if osteophytes and joint space narrowing are not present, another disorder should be considered.

The earliest sign of AVN is a joint effusion. This often is not radiographically visible or is so nonspecific that is does not help with the diagnosis unless the clinical setting had already raised suspicion for AVN. The next sign for AVN is a patchy or mottled density (Fig. 6-51). In the knee this density increase can occur throughout an entire condyle, whereas in the hip it often involves the entire femoral head. Next, subchondral lucency develops that forms a thin line along the articular surface (Fig. 6-52). This lucent line has been described as being an early indicator for AVN when, in fact, it is a late finding. Also, the lucent

FIGURE 6-51 **Early avascular necrosis of the hip.** Patchy sclerosis is present throughout the femoral head in this patient with a renal transplant and avascular necrosis of the right hip. No subchondral lucency or articular surface irregularity in the weight-bearing region is yet present with the exception of a small cortical irregularity seen laterally.

line stage is often not present in the evolution of AVN. Therefore, using the lucent line as one of the main criteria for AVN can lead to missing early findings or missing the diagnosis completely. I would estimate that I see a lucent line in only 20% or fewer of the cases of AVN in our hospital.

The final sign in AVN is collapse of the articular surface and joint fragmentation (Fig. 6-53). I must stress that these changes all occur on only one side of a joint, which makes for an easy diagnosis, because almost everything else around joints involves both sides.

MRI examination plays a valuable role in the early diagnosis of AVN throughout the skeletal system but especially in the hip, where it is more sensitive than even radionuclide scans. The use of MRI in AVN of the hip is discussed more fully in Chapter 13.

A form of AVN that is smaller and more focal than that just described is osteochondritis dissecans. For whatever reasons, the term osteochondritis dissecans has been replaced by the term osteochondral lesion (OCL). Perhaps the absence of true desiccation forced true academicians to choose a more acceptable term—I wish they'd just stick to one term, whether it's technically right or wrong! It is thought to be caused by trauma, although many believe that it is primarily idiopathic. It is most commonly found in the knee at the medial femoral condyle (Fig. 6-54), but it also is seen frequently in the dome of the talus (Fig. 6-55)

FIGURE 6-52 **Avascular necrosis of the hip.** Definite subchondral lucency (*arrows*) is seen in the weight-bearing portion of this hip with avascular necrosis. Patchy sclerosis throughout the femoral head is also noted.

FIGURE 6-53 **Avascular necrosis of the shoulder.** Articular surface collapse is present in this shoulder with long-standing avascular necrosis. Dense bony sclerosis is also present.

FIGURE 6-54 Osteochondral lesion (OCL). A small focal area of avascular necrosis in the medial condyle of the femur *(black arrows)* is present, which is an OCL. Part of the area of avascular necrosis has shed a bony fragment *(white arrow)* that is loose in the joint and is known as a joint mouse.

and occasionally in the capitellum (Fig. 6-56). Osteochondritis dissecans, oops, I mean an OCL, often leads to a small fragment of bone being sloughed off and becoming a free fragment in the joint—a "joint mouse" (see Fig. 6-54).

AVN is one of the disorders around joints in which subchondral cysts or "geodes" can occur. It is the only one of the four disorders (rheumatoid arthritis, DJD, and CPPD being the others) that can have an essentially normal joint and have a geode (Fig. 6-57). The other abnormalities will have joint space narrowing and/or osteophytes, osteoporosis, chondrocalcinosis, or other findings.

A host of names have been ascribed to epiphyseal AVN, usually with the eponym being the first person to describe the disorder. These are thought to be idiopathic for the most part but can also occur secondary to trauma. A few of the more common bones involved are the following: the carpal lunate (Kienböck's malacia [Fig. 6-58]); the tarsal navicular (Köhler's bone disease [Fig. 6-59]); the metatarsal heads (Freiberg's infraction [Fig. 6-60]); the femoral head (Legg-Perthes); the ring apophyses of the spine (Scheuermann's disease [Fig. 6-61]); and the tibial tubercle (Osgood-Schlatter disease, also called surfer's knees).

FIGURE 6-55 Osteochondral lesion (OCL) of the talus. A focal area of avascular necrosis in the talus as seen here *(arrows)* is called an OCL. The talus is the second most common site after the knee and, as in the knee, can cause a joint mouse or loose body in the joint.

FIGURE 6-56 Osteochondral lesion (OCL) of the elbow. The third most common site for an OCL is in the capitellum of the elbow. The faint lucency seen in this capitellum *(arrows)* was at first believed to be a chondroblastoma or an area of infection.

FIGURE 6-57 Geode in the hip. A large cystic lesion (*arrows*) is seen in this patient with avascular necrosis of the hip. Note the adjacent patchy sclerosis indicative of avascular necrosis. A subchondral cyst or geode should be considered any time a lytic lesion is found around a joint.

FIGURE 6-59 Köhler's bone disease. Flattening and sclerosis of the tarsal navicular (*arrow*) in children is thought by many to be avascular necrosis and is called Köhler's bone disease. Others have found this to be an asymptomatic normal variant and believe that it is an incidental finding.

FIGURE 6-58 Kienböck's malacia. Avascular necrosis of the lunate, or Kienböck's malacia, is demonstrated in this patient. Note the increased density and partial fragmentation of the lunate.

FIGURE 6-60 Freiberg's infraction. Flattening, collapse, and sclerosis of the second metatarsal head, as seen in this patient, are typical of avascular necrosis or Freiberg's infraction. It can also involve the third or fourth metatarsal heads. Note the compensatory hypertrophy of the cortex of the second metatarsal, which is invariably found with this disorder.

FIGURE 6-61 **Scheuermann's disease.** Avascular necrosis of the apophyseal rings of the vertebral bodies is called Scheuermann's disease. Scheuermann originally described a painful kyphosis with multiple vertebral bodies involved. It is most commonly seen without kyphosis or pain and with only a few vertebral bodies involved.

REFERENCES

1. Forrester DM, Brown JC: The Radiology of Joint Disease, 3rd ed. Philadelphia, WB Saunders, 1987.
2. Brower AC: Arthritis in Black and White, 2nd ed. Philadelphia, WB Saunders, 1997.
3. Resnick D: Diagnosis of Bone and Joint Disorders, 4th ed. Philadelphia, WB Saunders, 2002.

CHAPTER 7

Metabolic Bone Disease

Most of the literature on metabolic bone disease is steeped in biochemistry, physiology, histology, internal medicine, and other arcane pursuits that can be quite confusing for a poor radiology resident who just wants a few pearls and illustrations. Frankly, it's a tough topic. I will, by necessity, keep it simple; but this is an important topic about which every radiologist should have at least a superficial fund of knowledge. I have excluded disorders such as pseudo- and pseudo-pseudo-hypoparathyroidism that are unlikely to be seen, and I have tried to cover the more commonly seen disorders.

OSTEOPOROSIS

Osteoporosis is diminished bone quantity in which the bone is otherwise normal. This contrasts with osteomalacia, in which the bone quantity is normal but the bone itself is abnormal in that it is not normally mineralized. Osteomalacia results in excess nonmineralized osteoid. It is not possible in most cases to distinguish between osteoporosis and osteomalacia on plain films.

There are a myriad of causes of osteoporosis, the most common of which is senile osteoporosis, or osteoporosis of aging. This is seen most commonly in postmenopausal women and is a major public health concern because of the increase of spinal and hip fractures in this patient population. Another name for this type of osteoporosis is primary osteoporosis.

Secondary osteoporosis implies that an underlying disorder, such as thyrotoxicosis or renal disease, has caused the osteoporosis. Only about 5% of osteoporosis cases have an underlying cause. The differential diagnosis for secondary osteoporosis is quite long and probably should not be memorized, because one cannot even be sure if it is osteoporosis or osteomalacia on the basis of the

plain films. Therefore, the differential for presumed osteoporosis would have to include the causes of osteomalacia. The list gets too long to be of any real help to anyone.

The main radiographic finding in osteoporosis is thinning of the cortex. This is best demonstrated in the second metacarpal at the mid-diaphysis (Figs. 7-1 and 7-2). The normal metacarpal cortical thickening should be approximately one fourth to one third the thickness of the metacarpal (Fig. 7-3). In osteoporosis, this cortical thickness is decreased. The metacarpal cortex (and all bony cortices, for that matter) decreases normally with age and is less for women than for men of the same age. Several tables have been published that give the normal metacarpal cortical measurement, with age and sex adjustments to allow determination of normal. Unfortunately, these tables only determine the mineralization of the peripheral skeleton and do not seem to correlate to whether spinal or hip fractures will occur.

Measurement of the axial bone mineral content can be done by one of several methods that use computed tomography (CT) to assess the bone quantity in the spine. There is much debate over which method is superior and even whether knowing the bone mineral content is clinically helpful, because just knowing the age and sex of the patient is fairly accurate for predicting the bone mass quantity. Many experts say that knowing the axial bone mineral measurement does not help to predict which patients are at risk for spinal and hip fractures.

Exercise and proper diet (whatever that is) seem to help delay the onset of primary osteoporosis as much as anything. Calcium additives alone have not been shown to reverse the process of primary osteoporosis. Estrogen therapy has been found to be beneficial in delaying primary osteoporosis but is controversial in regards to its side effects. If it is

FIGURE 7-1 Mild osteoporosis. Mild cortical narrowing (*arrows*) at the mid-second metacarpal is noted in this patient with renal osteodystrophy. Note the calcification around the first metacarpophalangeal joint. Compare this cortical width with that of the normal width in Figure 7-3.

FIGURE 7-2 Marked osteoporosis. Marked cortical narrowing (*arrows*) of the mid-second metacarpal cortex is present in this patient with severe osteoporosis. Also note the intracortical tunneling, which occurs with more rapid forms of osteoporosis.

inevitable and cannot be treated in most cases, why go to a huge expense to diagnose it? That's one of the reasons this is a controversial topic.[1]

Because we cannot accurately give the causes of osteoporosis by looking at a radiograph and cannot even differentiate it from osteomalacia, it is a topic that is frustrating for many radiologists to deal with. Most of us would rather comment on something we can give a diagnosis on or at least a short differential. In general, when decreased bone mass is present on a radiograph, the odds are that osteoporosis is present. However, because the disease process could just as easily be osteomalacia, it is recommended that the term "osteopenia" be used. This is a generic term that includes both osteoporosis and osteomalacia. When used it also implies that the observer knows he or she cannot separate the two entities and is an educated person. It is radiographically correct but perhaps a bit pretentious.

A type of osteoporosis that can be seen in a patient of any age is disuse osteoporosis. It results from immobilization from any cause, most commonly after treatment of a fracture. The radiographic appearance of disuse osteoporosis is different from senile osteoporosis in that it occurs somewhat more rapidly and gives the bone a patchy

or even a permeative appearance (Fig. 7-4). This is from the osteocytic resorption in the cortex, causing intracortical holes. If allowed to continue with disuse, the bone would resemble any bone with marked osteoporosis (i.e., severe cortical thinning).

Occasionally, aggressive osteoporosis from disuse can mimic a permeative lesion, such as a Ewing's sarcoma or multiple myeloma, because of the severe cortical patchy or permeative pattern that projects over the medullary space and resembles a medullary permeative process (Fig. 7-5). The way to differentiate a true intramedullary permeative process from an intracortical process such as osteoporosis is to observe the cortex and see if it is solid or riddled with holes (Fig. 7-6). If it is solid, you can assume the permeative process is emanating from the medullary space (Fig. 7-7); if it has multiple small holes, you have to assume the permeative pattern is from the cortical process. I call a permeative appearance that is secondary to cortical holes a pseudopermeative process to distinguish it from a true permeative process.

Another cause for a pseudopermeative process is a hemangioma. It can cause cortical holes in two ways: from focal increased blood flow or hyperemia, causing focal osteoporosis, or by the blood

FIGURE 7-3 **Normal mineralization.** Note the cortical width (*arrows*) of the mid-second metacarpal in this patient with normal mineralization. The width of the cortex is easily greater than one third of the total width of the metacarpal.

FIGURE 7-4 **Aggressive osteoporosis.** A diffuse permeative pattern throughout the proximal femur is noted in this patient, who has recently had an amputation. Note that the cortices are riddled with holes, which would indicate that this is not a true intramedullary process but an intracortical process. This is distinctive for aggressive osteoporosis and causes a pseudopermeative pattern that can be mistaken for a more sinister process.

vessels themselves tunneling through the cortex (Figs. 7-8 and 7-9). I have seen more than one hemangioma operated on inadvertently because the lesion was thought to be a Ewing's sarcoma—they bleed a lot.

Radiotherapy can cause cortical holes in bone and mimic a permeative pattern (Fig. 7-10). These holes are often large and would not be confused with a true permeative process, but they can be small and cause confusion.

If a permeative pattern is seen in bone, the differential is usually an aggressive process such as Ewing's sarcoma, infection, or eosinophilic granuloma in a young person or multiple myeloma, metastatic carcinomatosis, or primary lymphoma of bone in an older patient. If, however, the permeative pattern is seen to be a result of cortical holes (i.e., a pseudopermeative pattern), the differential is considerably kinder: aggressive osteoporosis, hemangioma, or radiation changes. This differential does not arise often but is useful when it does occur.[2]

OSTEOMALACIA

As mentioned earlier, osteomalacia is the result of too much nonmineralized osteoid. There are many causes for osteomalacia, with the most common currently being renal osteodystrophy. The radiographic findings are almost identical to those of osteoporosis, and for the most part the two disorders are indistinguishable. The only findings that are distinctive for osteomalacia are Looser's zone fractures, which are fractures through large osteoid seams (Fig. 7-11). They are extremely uncommon but tend to occur in the pelvis and scapula.

In children, osteomalacia is called rickets. It causes the epiphyses to become flared and irregular, and the long bones undergo bending from the bone softening (Fig. 7-12). As in adults, the most common cause is renal disease, although other causes, such as biliary disease and dietary insufficiencies, are seen.

HYPERPARATHYROIDISM

Hyperparathyroidism (HPT) occurs from excess parathyroid hormone (PTH). PTH causes osteoclastic

FIGURE 7-5 **Cortical holes in osteoporosis.** This patient experienced a stroke and has aggressive osteoporosis secondary to disuse. What appears to be a diffuse permeative pattern throughout the humerus is noted, on closer inspection, to be cortical holes, which, in this case, are caused by the aggressive osteoporosis. This type of pattern, unfortunately, often leads to a biopsy to rule out multiple myeloma or other round cell tumors.

FIGURE 7-6 **Schematic of cortical holes.** This schematic of a permeative lesion *(A)* shows how only the endosteum is affected with the bulk of the cortex spared. A pseudopermeative lesion *(B)* has the entire cortex affected. Both processes will look permeative on a plain film; however, the true permeative process will have an uninvolved cortex.

resorption in bone, which leads to osteoporosis and osteomalacia. The most common cause is renal disease, which leads to secondary HPT. Secondary HPT is caused by the response of the parathyroids to hypocalcemia. Parathyroid adenomas and hyperplasia can cause primary HPT. Up to 40% of patients with primary HPT will demonstrate skeletal abnormalities radiographically.

The radiographic sign that is pathognomonic for HPT is subperiosteal bone resorption. It is seen most commonly on the radial aspect of the middle phalanges of the hand (Fig. 7-13) but can be seen in any long bone in the body. It is commonly seen on the medial aspect of the proximal tibia (Fig. 7-14), in the distal clavicles, and in the sacroiliac (SI) joints, where it resembles bilateral sacroiliitis (Fig. 7-15).

Other radiographic findings include osteosclerosis, usually diffuse, but often involving the spine in a manner resembling the stripes on rugby jerseys, hence the name "rugger jersey spine" (Fig. 7-16). Brown tumors are cystic lesions that are often expansile and aggressive in appearance (Fig. 7-17). They were once said to be more common in primary HPT but are seen most commonly associated with secondary HPT today because of the overwhelming preponderance of patients with secondary as compared with primary disease. They are only rarely seen without other evidence of HPT, such as subperiosteal resorption; therefore, I will not include a brown tumor in my differential diagnosis of a cystic lesion if the remainder of the bones are normal. A brown tumor can have a variety of appearances; therefore, the only thing characteristic about it is that it is associated with subperiosteal bone resorption.

PTH can have an accelerating effect on bone that is undergoing slow change. In degenerative joint disease, especially in the spine, PTH can cause the

FIGURE 7-7 **Pathologic fracture in multiple myeloma.** This patient has multiple myeloma, which has caused a diffuse permeative pattern throughout his pelvis. He suffered an intertrochanteric fracture of his left hip (*curved arrow*), which was believed to be either caused by the osteoporosis present or by the infiltration of myeloma in this region. If myeloma were the cause of the fracture, radiation treatment before pinning was being considered. If, however, the fracture were caused by osteoporosis, radiation would not be given. A close look at the cortex in the proximal third of the femur (*straight arrow*) showed that it is not riddled with holes as it would be with osteoporosis; therefore, this was believed to be a pathologic fracture in an area of myeloma involvement. Surgery confirmed this.

affected joint or disc space to mimic infection (Fig. 7-18). PTH makes the usually sclerotic endplates fuzzy and eroded, and the narrowed disc space, which is a part of the degenerative disc disease, makes infection seem more likely. Therefore, patients with renal disease who have a presumed radiographic diagnosis of joint or disc space infection should not have an aspiration or biopsy unless strong clinical suspicion for infection is present.

How often is HPT present without subperiosteal resorption also being present? Not often, but it undoubtedly occurs. I am willing to miss all the cases of HPT that do not have associated subperiosteal resorption.

FIGURE 7-8 **Hemangioma.** Cortical holes of varying sizes are seen throughout the tibia in this patient with a large hemangioma of the tibia. Also note the phleboliths present in the soft tissues (*arrows*). It would be unlikely for osteoporosis to cause cortical holes of this size.

What causes osteosclerosis in HPT? No one really knows. Several theories have evolved to explain it, but none are totally satisfactory and are best left to others to worry about.

OSTEOSCLEROSIS

The radiographic finding of diffuse increased bone density—osteosclerosis—is somewhat uncommon, yet every radiologist must have a differential diagnosis for this process. Fortunately, it is a rather short differential, and there are criteria to narrow down the list of possibilities.

Dealing with the differential diagnosis for osteosclerosis is a three-step process. First, one must recognize that the bones are truly increased in density. This sounds straightforward enough but is, in fact, often difficult to do. Technical factors can easily alter the apparent bone density and be misleading. Second, once it is determined that diffuse osteosclerosis is present, one merely has to list the disease entities that could be responsible. This is the easiest step because it merely requires memorization. I will supply a mnemonic to help your memory. Lastly, one must look for radiographic findings that are specific for each disorder to rule them out or in so as to narrow down the list of

FIGURE 7-9 **Hemangioma**. A permeative pattern in the distal tibia was seen in this child with pain and an associated soft tissue mass. It was presumed to be a Ewing's sarcoma, and a biopsy was done with great loss of blood. A close examination of the cortex shows that the medial aspect is diffusely riddled with cortical holes, as compared with the lateral aspect. Although a Ewing's sarcoma could perhaps do this, one would expect diffuse periostitis to be present with cortical involvement of this extent.

FIGURE 7-10 **Osteonecrosis secondary to radiation**. Radiation to the femur for a soft tissue sarcoma some years before this plain film has caused large cortical holes throughout the femur. It is not likely that cortical holes of this size would be caused by osteoporosis, but they could be caused by a hemangioma.

possibilities. The list of diseases that cause diffuse osteosclerosis is different with each textbook that you read. There are many disorders that have been reported to cause osteosclerosis, but you only need a list that is correct 95 to 98% of the time. Nobody expects you to include the one reported case of hunchback midget whale syndrome in your list. If you absolutely cannot bear the thought of leaving out a possibility in your differential diagnosis, you might as well just give your clinician the index from Resnick's book[3]—it will be all-inclusive but not really useful to the clinician (not to imply that Resnick's book is not useful—it is the Bible for bone radiologists).

The entities I include in the differential for diffuse osteosclerosis are the following:

- renal osteodystrophy
- sickle cell disease
- myelofibrosis
- osteopetrosis
- pyknodysostosis
- metastatic carcinoma
- mastocytosis
- Paget's disease
- athletes
- fluorosis

The mnemonic I use to remember them is "Regular sex makes occasional perversions much more pleasurable and fantastic." Hey, it's not a great mnemonic, but in the 21st century it's not politically correct to be ribald, vulgar, off-color, coarse, crude, erotic, lewd, or even, sometimes, funny. If you want a filthy mnemonic, make up your own, you insensitive pervert.

I will cover each of these topics in generalities, trying to point out the features of each that you should look for to allow including or excluding them from the differential. A nice feature of this mnemonic is it lists the entities in their order of frequency. Not that osteopetrosis is more common than Paget's or metastatic disease (mets), but it's more common to see osteopetrosis than either Paget's or mets presenting as diffuse bony sclerosis.

FIGURE 7-11   Looser's zone fractures in osteomalacia. A horizontal fracture of the tibia and the fibula is present in this child with osteomalacia (rickets). Fractures of this type are called Looser's zone fractures and are virtually pathognomonic for osteomalacia; however, they are rarely seen.

FIGURE 7-12   Rickets. Osteomalacia in children causes fraying and splaying of the epiphyses, as well as bending of the bone secondary to bone softening. This condition has been termed rickets and is most commonly seen in renal disease.

Renal Osteodystrophy.   Anything that causes HPT can cause osteosclerosis, but renal disease is far and away the biggest offender. As mentioned previously, the *sine qua non* of renal osteodystrophy is subperiosteal bone resorption, seen earliest and most reliably at the radial aspect of the middle phalanges of the hands. Without this finding I will not entertain osteosclerosis being caused by renal disease. About 10 to 20% of patients with renal osteodystrophy will exhibit osteosclerosis, and the reasons for it are unknown.

Sickle Cell Disease.   Like renal osteodystrophy, the reason for dense bones to occur in sickle cell disease is unknown. It occurs in only a small percentage of patients. Additional signs to look for are bone infarcts and H-shaped or stepoff deformities of the vertebral body end-plates (Fig. 7-19). These are also called "fish vertebrae" after their similarity to the vertebrae found in fish.

Myelofibrosis.   Also called agnogenic myeloid metaplasia, myelofibrosis is a disease caused by progressive fibrosis of the marrow in patients older than 50 years. It leads to anemia with splenomegaly and extramedullary hematopoiesis. Whenever osteosclerosis is seen in a patient older than 50 years, a search for a large spleen and extramedullary hematopoiesis should be made (Fig. 7-20).

Osteopetrosis.   Osteopetrosis is a rare hereditary abnormality that results in extremely dense

FIGURE 7-13   Hyperparathyroidism.   Subperiosteal bone resorption is noted along the radial aspect of the middle phalanges (*arrows*), which is pathognomonic for hyperparathyroidism. The lytic lesion seen in the distal part of the middle phalanx (*curved arrow*) is either a brown tumor or a geode.

Figure 7-14 Hyperparathyroidism. Subperiosteal bone resorption is noted along the medial aspect of the proximal tibias *(arrows)*, which is a characteristic location. This is pathognomonic for hyperparathyroidism.

F igure **7-15 Hyperparathyroidism with sacroiliac (SI) joint subperiosteal erosion.** Bilateral SI joint widening and erosions can be seen in this patient with renal disease. This is caused by subperiosteal resorption and is a frequent finding in children with hyperparathyroidism.

bones throughout the skeleton (Fig. 7-21). There is a congenita and a tarda form with different degrees of severity in each. It is not so rare that you will never see a case; therefore, I include it in this differential list. A characteristic finding is the "bone-in-bone" appearance often seen in the vertebral bodies, in which the vertebrae have a small replica of the vertebral body inside the normal one (Fig. 7-22). Also characteristic is the "sandwich

F igure **7-16 Hyperparathyroidism.** Sclerotic bands are seen along the vertebral body end-plates. This has been termed a "rugger jersey spine" and is characteristic for hyperparathyroidism. Note how the sclerotic bands in the rugger jersey spine such as this are much less distinct and more fuzzy than the sclerotic bands seen in osteopetrosis in Figure 7-23.

FIGURE 7-17 **Hyperparathyroidism.** Lytic lesions are seen in the fifth metacarpal and at the base of the fourth proximal phalanx in this patient with hyperparathyroidism. Note the subperiosteal bone resorption seen along the radial aspect of the middle phalanges (*arrows*). Any cystic lesion in a patient with hyperparathyroidism must be considered a brown tumor until proven otherwise.

vertebrae," in which the end-plates are densely sclerotic, giving the appearance of a sandwich (Fig. 7-23). These findings do not have to be present to make the diagnosis, but their absence makes the diagnosis less likely.

Pyknodysostosis. Pyknodysostosis is the other congenital abnormality with dense bones that should be considered in the differential diagnosis for osteosclerosis. Like osteopetrosis, it is rare but is seen from time to time in busy radiology practices. These patients are typically short and have hypoplastic mandibles. The distinguishing radiographic finding that is essentially pathognomonic is that the distal phalanges often have the appearance of chalk that has been put into a pencil sharpener—they are pointed and dense (Fig. 7-24). Nothing else does this, but unfortunately pyknodysostosis does not do this in every case. Another name for this disorder is Toulouse-Lautrec syndrome; this famous artist was apparently afflicted with pyknodysostosis.

Metastatic Carcinoma. Only rarely will diffuse metastatic carcinoma cause a problem in diagnosis. I have seen only a handful of cases in which diffuse mets mimicked diffuse osteosclerosis, and in every case the primary tumor was prostate or breast carcinoma. If cortical destruction or a lytic component is present, the differential diagnosis is simplified, therefore these should be searched for.

Mastocytosis. Mastocytosis is another rare disorder that can cause uniform increased bone density. Unfortunately, there are no other plain film findings that might help with the diagnosis. These patients have thickened small-bowel folds with nodules, but of course to see them an upper gastrointestinal contrast study must be performed (Fig. 7-25). Mastocytosis is rare enough that you might be justified in leaving it out of your differential—you won't miss many, but it messes up the mnemonic.

Paget's Disease. Although Paget's disease in bone is common, diffuse Paget's disease that could be confused with one of the other diseases in the differential diagnosis of generalized osteosclerosis is rare—I have seen only one or two cases ever. Paget's disease classically causes bony enlargement (Fig. 7-26), but this is not always present. It occurs most commonly in the pelvis (Fig. 7-27), where it has been said the iliopectineal line on the pelvic brim must be thickened if Paget's disease is present. In fact, the iliopectineal line is usually, but not always, thickened. Paget's disease can occur in any bone in the body, including the smaller bones of the hands and feet (Fig. 7-28). It has been spread through the teaching files of many institutions (I have seen many statements in teaching files that have never made the literature that have served me well and others that have misled me) that the fibula is the only bone that Paget's never affects. I must agree that the fibula is usually spared—even with profound disease all around it—but I have certainly seen exceptions to this rule.

Three distinct phases are radiographically visible in Paget's disease: a lytic phase, a sclerotic phase, and a mixed lytic-sclerotic phase (Fig. 7-29). The lytic phase often has a sharp leading edge, called a "flame-shaped" or "blade of grass" leading edge. In a long bone, with the sole exception being the tibia, Paget's disease always starts at the end of the bone; therefore, if a lesion is present in the middle of a long bone and does not extend to either end, you can safely exclude Paget's disease.

So why is Paget's disease in this differential if it so rarely fits? Good question. You can probably safely leave it out without missing too many cases, but it's good to at least think about, because it is so readily diagnosed once you do think of it. Also, it does occasionally involve a large area, such as the entire pelvis, and makes the observer think that the entire skeleton might be involved.

When Paget's disease involves the skull it often causes thickening of the base of the skull (Fig. 7-30), whereas entities that cause osteoscle-

FIGURE 7-18   Parathyroid hormone discitis. *A,* A lateral plain film of the lumbar spine reveals disc space narrowing with erosion of the end-plates at the L2-3 level *(arrow).* This is a typical appearance of disc infection. *B,* A sagittal T1-weighted image of the lumbar spine reveals disc space narrowing and low signal extending into the end-plates and vertebral bodies adjacent to the L2-3 disc. *C,* A T2-weighted image shows high signal in the L2-3 disc and in the tissue extending into the vertebral bodies. This is the classic magnetic resonance imaging appearance of disc infection with involvement of the vertebral bodies. However, this patient has renal osteodystrophy, and hyperparathyroidism can cause changes in the joints and the disc spaces identical to infection. Clinical correlation must be used to avoid an unnecessary biopsy.

rosis due to marrow disease (sickle cell and myelofibrosis) will spare the base of the skull because it contains no marrow. This point is best illustrated by thalassemia in which the calvarium is thickened by marrow hyperplasia, whereas the base of the skull is spared (Fig. 7-31).

Athletes.   I see radiographs on professional athletes quite often and continue to be impressed by the degree of increased cortical thickness these people possess. No question about it: increased stress causes hypertrophy of bone, as well as of muscle. I see radiologists routinely question the presence of diffuse increased bone density in this set of patients, enough so that I have added normal athletes to my differential diagnosis for osteosclerosis.

Fluorosis.   Fluorosis is another rare disorder that could probably be left off the list without danger of missing too many cases. Fluorosis is usually a result of chronic intake in certain areas that have large amounts of fluoride present in the drinking water. It can also be a result of long-term therapy

FIGURE 7-21 **Osteopetrosis**. Diffuse bony sclerosis is present throughout the skeleton in this patient with osteopetrosis.

FIGURE 7-19 **Sickle cell disease**. Stepoff deformities are seen in the end-plates of multiple vertebral bodies in this patient with sickle cell disease. Although the bones do not show osteosclerosis, the visible trabeculae are somewhat coarsened. The stepoff deformities in the spine are characteristic for sickle cell disease. These are also called "fish vertebrae."

FIGURE 7-20 **Myelofibrosis**. Uniform increased bone density seen most prominently throughout the pelvis is present in this patient with myelofibrosis. Note the grossly enlarged spleen (*arrows*) and the opaque iron tablets (*curved arrow*), which are taken for the anemia often present in this disorder.

FIGURE 7-22 **Osteopetrosis**. A "bone-in-bone" appearance is present in the vertebral bodies in this patient with osteopetrosis. This is often seen in osteopetrosis and is occasionally seen in other disorders.

FIGURE 7-23 **Osteopetrosis.** "Sandwich vertebrae" are seen in the vertebral bodies in this patient with osteopetrosis. This is virtually pathognomonic for osteopetrosis when present and should not be confused with the ill-defined bands of sclerosis seen in the rugger jersey spine of hyperparathyroidism.

FIGURE 7-24 **Pyknodysostosis.** Dense sclerosis is seen throughout the hand in this patient with pyknodysostosis. A pathognomonic finding is seen in the distal phalanges, where the tufts are absent and the phalanges are pointed and sclerotic.

with sodium fluoride for osteoporosis. A radiographic finding that patients with fluorosis often have is ligamentous calcification. If I have a patient with dense bones and no ligamentous calcifications, I will put fluorosis lower on the list but not eliminate it. If ligamentous calcifications are present, it will go to the top of the list. Calcification of the sacrotuberous ligament is said to be characteristic for fluorosis.

CONCLUSION

There are other categories of disease that could be covered in a chapter on metabolic bone disease, but most of the remaining disorders are exceedingly rare and not likely to be seen by most radiologists on a routine basis. Excellent textbooks are available for additional details on the diseases I have mentioned and for learning about the less common entities.

FIGURE 7-25 **Mastocytosis.** Uniform dense bones are noted throughout the pelvis in this patient with mastocytosis. Note the thickened small-bowel folds with nodules (*arrow*), which are often seen in mastocytosis.

FIGURE 7-26 **Paget's disease.** Dense sclerosis with bony overgrowth is seen in the L3 vertebral body in this patient with Paget's disease. The left L3 pedicle is particularly dense and overgrown.

FIGURE 7-28 **Paget's disease.** Dense sclerosis of the capitate *(arrow)* is seen in this patient. Although no definite bony overgrowth is appreciated, it is not unusual for Paget's disease to affect a single bone uniformly such as this.

FIGURE 7-27 **Paget's disease.** Dense bony sclerosis with some bony enlargement is seen throughout the left pelvis and proximal femur. Note the thickening of the iliopectineal line on the left side *(arrow)* as compared with the right side.

FIGURE 7-31 **Thalassemia.** This patient with thalassemia has marked thickening of the calvarium with sparing of the base of the skull.

REFERENCES

1. Hall FM: Bone-mineral screening for osteoporosis. Opinion. AJR 1987;149:120-122.
2. Helms C, Munk P: Pseudopermeative skeletal lesions. Br J Radiol 1990;63:461-467.
3. Resnick D: Diagnosis of Bone and Joint Disorders, 4th ed. Philadelphia, WB Saunders, 2002.

FIGURE 7-29 **Paget's disease.** A "flame-shaped" or "blade of grass" appearance is seen in the distal tibia (*arrow*) in this patient with Paget's disease of the tibia. The sclerotic phase of Paget's disease is seen in the mid-tibia in this patient, whereas the proximal tibia has an area of apparent cortical destruction (*curved arrow*), which is suspicious for sarcomatous degeneration.

FIGURE 7-30 **Paget's disease.** This patient with Paget's disease shows marked thickening of the base of the skull on this lateral skull film.

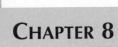

CHAPTER 8

Miscellaneous Conditions

There are a host of bony conditions, diseases, and syndromes that do not fit conveniently into any of the preceding chapters, but they should be given some mention in an attempted overview of musculoskeletal radiology. Many of these are simply "Aunt Minnies" and only require you to have seen them once or twice to recognize them. I have severely limited the things I have included in this chapter—it could easily have had dozens of other entities, but none are common. Besides, I need to have something to add in future editions. These are listed alphabetically for lack of a more scientific basis.

ACHONDROPLASIA

The most common cause of dwarfism is achondroplasia, a congenital, hereditary disease of failure of endochondral bone formation. The femurs and humeri are more profoundly affected than the other long bones, although the entire skeleton is abnormal. The spine typically has narrowing of the interpedicular distances in a caudal direction (Fig. 8-1), the opposite of normal where the interpedicular distances get progressively wider as one proceeds down the spine. I know of no other entity that has narrowing of the interpedicular distance, and I have never seen a case of achondroplasia without this narrowing. The long bones are short but have normal width, giving them a thick appearance.

AVASCULAR NECROSIS

The term avascular necrosis (AVN), also called osteonecrosis, refers to the lack of blood supply with subsequent bone death and ensuing bony collapse in an articular surface. The cause of AVN is an extensive differential that most commonly includes trauma, steroids, aspirin, sickle cell dis-

ease, collagen vascular diseases, alcoholism, and idiopathic origins (Table 8-1).[1] The radiographic appearance ranges from patchy sclerosis (Fig. 8-2A) to articular surface collapse and fragmentation (Fig. 8-3). Just before collapse, a subchondral lucency is occasionally seen (Fig. 8-4); however, this is a late and inconstant sign of AVN. Magnetic resonance imaging (MRI) is extremely valuable in demonstrating the presence and extent of AVN (see Fig. 8-2B and C) even when plain films are apparently normal. MRI is currently considered to be the most efficacious way to evaluate a joint for AVN.[2] It is useful not only in AVN of the hips but also of the knee, wrist, foot, and ankle.

ENGELMANN'S DISEASE

Also known as diaphyseal dysplasia, Engelmann's disease is a congenital disorder that is manifested by diaphyseal cortical thickening that primarily involves the long bones, particularly the lower extremity (Fig. 8-5). Although it can be asymptomatic and incidental, these children can have a painful, waddling gait, and it can progress dramatically causing severe medullary encroachment with subsequent anemia.

HYPERTROPHIC PULMONARY OSTEOARTHROPATHY

Hypertrophic pulmonary osteoarthropathy (HPO) is manifested by clubbing of the fingers and periostitis, usually in the upper and lower extremities (Fig. 8-6), which may or may not be associated with bone pain. It is most commonly seen in patients with lung cancer, but many other etiologic factors have been reported, including bronchiectasis, gastrointestinal disorders, and liver disease. The actual mechanism of formation of periostitis secondary to a distant malignancy or other process

155

FIGURE 8-1   Achondroplasia. An anteroposterior plain film of the spine in this patient with achondroplasia demonstrates narrowing of the interpedicular distance (*arrows*) in a caudal direction, which is characteristic of this disorder. Ordinarily, the interpedicular distance widens in each vertebra in a caudal direction.

is unknown. The differential diagnosis for periostitis in a long bone without an underlying bony abnormality would include HPO, venous stasis, thyroid acropachy, pachydermoperiostosis, and trauma (Table 8-2).

MELORHEOSTOSIS

Melorheostosis is a rare, idiopathic disorder characterized by thickened cortical new bone that accumulates near the ends of long bones, usually only on one side of the bone, and has an appearance likened to "dripping candle wax" (Fig. 8-7). It can affect several adjacent bones and can be symptomatic. Many feel there is some relation or overlap among melorheostosis, osteopathia striata, and osteopoikilosis (mentioned later in this chapter), all of which present with varying patterns of increased cortical bone.

TABLE 8-1   **Common Causes of Avascular Necrosis**

Trauma	Collagen vascular diseases
Steroids	Alcoholism
Aspirin	Idiopathic
Sickle cell disease	

FIGURE 8-2   Avascular necrosis. *A,* A plain film of the hip in this patient with avascular necrosis (AVN) shows faint patchy sclerosis throughout the femoral head. This is a relatively early plain film finding for AVN. Coronal (*B*) and axial (*C*) MR images in the same patient, which are T1 weighted (TR, 500; TE, 28), show typical findings in AVN. Diffuse low signal in the right hip is noted, which indicates more extensive involvement than in the left. The left hip has a low-signal serpiginous rim (*arrow*), which is characteristic for AVN.

FIGURE 8-3   **Avascular necrosis (AVN).** An anteroposterior plain film of the shoulder reveals articular surface collapse in this patient who was treated with steroids for systemic lupus erythematosus. This is an advanced stage of AVN.

FIGURE 8-5   **Engelmann's disease.** An anteroposterior film of the femurs shows bilateral cortical thickening that is localized to the diaphyses.

FIGURE 8-4   **Avascular necrosis (AVN).** An anteroposterior frog-leg lateral view of the hip in this patient with sickle cell disease shows a subchondral lucency (*arrows*) and patchy sclerosis in the femoral head, indicative of AVN. This is a relatively advanced stage of AVN. The subchondral lucency is often better demonstrated with the frog-leg lateral view.

FIGURE 8-6   **Hypertrophic pulmonary osteoarthropathy (HPO).** Periostitis can be seen along the shafts of the distal tibia and fibula (*arrows*) in this patient with bronchogenic carcinoma and leg pain. This is characteristic for HPO.

TABLE 8-2	Periostitis without Underlying Bony Lesion
Trauma	Venous stasis
Hypertrophic pulmonary osteoarthropathy	Thyroid acropachy
	Pachydermoperiostosis

MUCOPOLYSACCHARIDOSES (MORQUIO'S, HURLER'S, AND HUNTER'S SYNDROMES)

The mucopolysaccharidoses are a group of inherited diseases characterized by abnormal storage and excretion in the urine of various mucopolysaccharides such as keratan sulfate (Morquio's syndrome) and heparan sulfate (Hurler's syndrome). These patients have short stature, primarily from shortened spines, and characteristic plain film findings. In the spine, patients with Morquio's syndrome have platyspondyly (generalized flattening of the verte-bral bodies) with a central anterior projection or "beak" off of the vertebral body as viewed on a lateral plain film (Fig. 8-8). Hurler's and Hunter's syndromes show platyspondyly with a "beak" that is anteroinferiorly positioned (Fig. 8-9). The pelvis in these disorders is similar in appearance to that of achondroplasty with wide, flared iliac wings and broad femoral necks. A characteristic finding in the hands is a pointed proximal fifth metacarpal base that has a notch appearance to the ulnar aspect (Fig. 8-10).

MULTIPLE HEREDITARY EXOSTOSES

Also known as diaphyseal aclasia, multiple hereditary exostoses is a not uncommon hereditary disorder that seems to affect multiple members of a family with multiple osteochondromas, or exostoses. An osteochondroma is a cartilage-capped bone outgrowth, which may be pedunculated or sessile in appearance. In the multiple hereditary form, the knees are virtually always involved (Fig. 8-11). The incidence of malignant degeneration in this population has been reported to be as high as 20%, but this is a gross overestimation with the actual incidence being probably less than 1%. As with solitary osteochondromas, the more axi-

FIGURE 8-7 **Melorheostosis.** Dense, wavy, new bone is seen adjacent to the lateral tibial cortex, which has a "dripping candle wax" appearance that is classic for melorheostosis. A similar pattern can be seen in the medial aspect of the distal femur.

FIGURE 8-8 **Morquio's syndrome.** A lateral plain film of the spine reveals a central "beak" or anterior bony projection off of the vertebral bodies in this patient with Morquio's syndrome.

FIGURE 8-9 **Hurler's syndrome.** A lateral plain film of the spine in this patient with Hurler's syndrome shows an inferiorly placed bony projection extending anteriorly off of the vertebral bodies (*arrow*).

FIGURE 8-11 **Multiple hereditary exostosis.** The knees are involved in virtually every case of multiple hereditary exostosis. They typically show not only multiple exostoses (*arrows*) but also marked undertubulation (widening) in the metaphyses.

ally situated lesions are more prone to undergo malignant degeneration, whereas the more peripheral lesions are less likely to do so. The proximal femurs are frequently involved and have a characteristic appearance (Fig. 8-12).

FIGURE 8-10 **Hurler's syndrome.** An anteroposterior plain film of the hand in this patient with Hurler's syndrome shows a notch (*arrow*) at the base of the fifth metacarpal, which is a characteristic finding in all of the mucopolysaccharidoses.

FIGURE 8-12 **Multiple hereditary exostosis.** The femoral necks are often involved in multiple hereditary exostosis. They will show undertubulation, as in this example, and usually have one or more exostoses (*arrows*). Note the involvement of the superior pubic rami and the symphysis.

OSTEOID OSTEOMA

The cause of osteoid osteoma is unknown. Is it an infection (bacterial or viral), a slow-growing tumor, a dessert topping? Nobody knows. It is a painful lesion that occurs almost exclusively in patients younger than 30 years that is treated successfully with surgical excision or, more commonly today, percutaneous radiofrequency ablation. Aspirin often gives dramatic relief of the pain and can be used for conservative treatment in lieu of surgery. A classic clinical picture for an osteoid osteoma is "night pain relieved by aspirin." However, many osteoid osteomas do not have this presentation, and most painful musculoskeletal lesions are worse at night and are relieved by aspirin; therefore, this can lead to confusion.

Radiographically, an osteoid osteoma is said to have a typical appearance, but, in fact, it has many different appearances, which can make diagnosis difficult.[3] The classically described radiographic appearance is a cortically based sclerotic lesion in a long bone that has a small lucency within it, which is called the nidus (Fig. 8-13A). It is the nidus that causes the pain and the surrounding reactive sclerosis. If the nidus is surgically removed or ablated percutaneously with radiofrequency, complete cessation of pain is the rule. Computed tomography (CT) and radionuclide bone scanning are often helpful in demonstrating the exact location of the nidus (see Fig. 8-13B and C).

If the nidus of an osteoid osteoma is located in the medullary rather than the cortical portion of a bone, or if it is located in a joint, there is much less reactive sclerosis present. This gives the lesion a different overall appearance than the more common cortical lesion in that it does not appear as sclerotic. Up to 80% of osteoid osteomas are located intracortically with the remainder being in the intramedullary part of a bone. Rarely, an osteoid osteoma will present in the periosteum causing tremendous periostitis.

The nidus itself is usually lucent but often develops some calcification within it. It then has the appearance of a sequestrum as is seen in osteomyelitis. If the nidus calcifies completely, it blends in with the surrounding sclerosis and cannot be seen on most radiographs. Therefore, the diagnosis of an osteoid osteoma in no way is dependent on seeing a nidus.

Because an osteoid osteoma resembles osteomyelitis, regardless of the appearance of the nidus, it can be difficult to differentiate the two radiographically. In fact, it cannot be done with plain films, CT scanning, or MRI. However, because the nidus is extremely vascular, it avidly accumulates radiopharmaceutical bone scanning agents. An osteoid osteoma will have an area of increased uptake corresponding to the area of reactive sclerosis, but, in addition, will demonstrate a second area of increased uptake corresponding to the nidus (Figs. 8-13 to 8-15). This has been termed the "double density" sign.[4] In contrast, osteomyelitis has a photopenic area corresponding to the plain film lucency, which represents an avas-cular focus of purulent material. The natural history of an osteoid osteoma is presumed to be spontaneous regression because they are rarely seen in patients older than 30 years.

OSTEOPATHIA STRIATA

Also known as Voorhoeve's disease, osteopathia striata is manifested by multiple 2- to 3-mm-thick linear bands of sclerotic bone aligned parallel to the long axis of a bone (Fig. 8-16). It usually affects multiple long bones and is asymptomatic; hence, it is usually an incidental finding.

OSTEOPOIKILOSIS

Osteopoikilosis is a hereditary, asymptomatic disorder that is usually an incidental finding of multiple small (3 to 10 mm) sclerotic bony densities affecting primarily the ends of long bones and the pelvis (Fig. 8-17). It has virtually no clinical significance other than that it can be confused for diffuse osteoblastic metastases.

PACHYDERMOPERIOSTOSIS

Pachydermoperiostosis is a rare, familial disease that is manifested by periostitis in the extremities, thickening of the skin of the extremities and face, and clubbing of the fingers. It seems to be more common in the African-American population. The periosteal reaction is similar to that of HPO (Fig. 8-18), but pachydermoperiostosis is rarely painful.

SARCOID

Sarcoidosis is a noncaseating granulomatous disease that primarily affects the lungs. When the musculoskeletal system is involved, the hands are mainly affected, with the spine and long bones only infrequently involved. Sarcoid causes a characteristic "lacelike" pattern of bony destruction in the hands (Fig. 8-19). Multiple phalanges are typically affected in either one or both hands. It is so radiographically characteristic that there is almost no differential diagnosis for this pattern.

SLIPPED CAPITAL FEMORAL EPIPHYSIS

The epiphysis of the femoral head (called the capital epiphysis) has a tendency to slip medially. This is seen primarily in young teenage boys who are overweight, although it can be seen in hyperparathyroidism or idiopathically. It can be identified on an anteroposterior view of the pelvis or hips by

FIGURE 8-13 **Osteoid osteoma.** *A*, An anteroposterior plain film of the femur in a child with hip pain shows an area of sclerosis medially near the lesser trochanter with a small lucency *(arrow)*, which is the nidus of an osteoid osteoma. Osteomyelitis could have this identical appearance. *B*, A radionuclide bone scan shows increased uptake in the proximal femur, which corresponds to the reactive new bone seen on the plain film. In addition, however, note the second smaller area of increased radionuclide uptake within the larger area *(arrow)*. This corresponds to the nidus itself. This pattern on a bone scan is called the double density sign. *C*, A CT scan of the femur shows the sclerosis medially and the lucent nidus *(arrow)* to better advantage. The CT and the bone scan give the surgeon a more precise anatomic location of the nidus than the plain film.

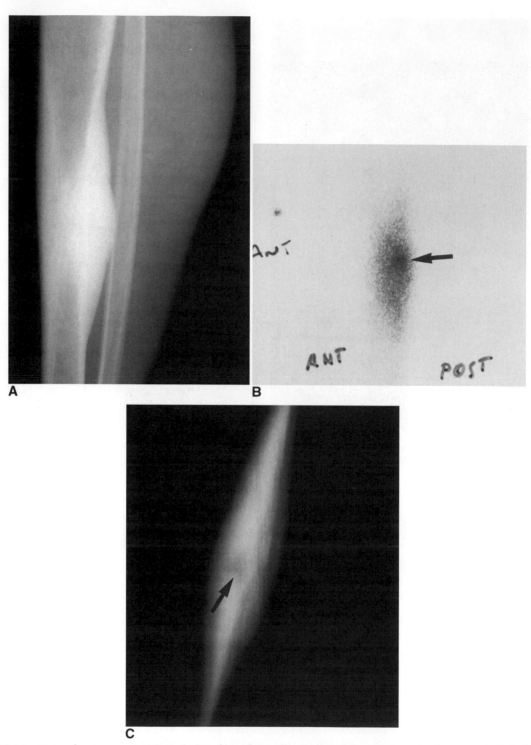

FIGURE 8-14   Osteoid osteoma. *A,* A lateral plain film of the tibia in this child with leg pain shows cortical thickening in the posterior diaphysis. No lucency in the sclerotic area could be identified. *B,* A radionuclide bone scan reveals uptake corresponding to the area of sclerosis in the tibia, with a more marked area of uptake centrally *(arrow),* which is the double density sign of an osteoid osteoma. *C,* The surgical specimen shows the nidus *(arrow)* as a faint lucency within the sclerotic bone.

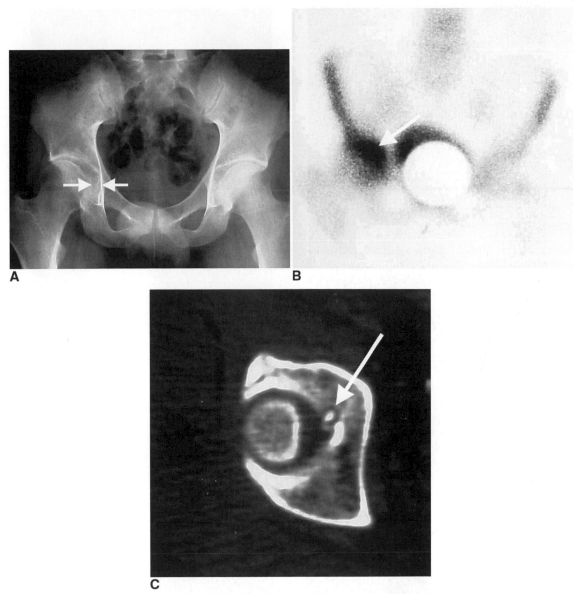

FIGURE 8-15 **Osteoid osteoma.** *A,* A plain film of the hips in this 24-year-old man with right hip pain shows a widened teardrop *(arrows)* measurement on the right as compared with the left. This indicates a joint effusion. No other abnormality was found; therefore, an aspiration arthrogram was performed to exclude infection. It was normal except for a joint effusion, which was culture negative. A radionuclide bone scan *(B)* was done to see if AVN or a stress fracture was the source of the pain. It revealed increased uptake throughout the acetabulum with a second area of increased uptake *(arrow)* corresponding to a double density sign. A CT scan *(C)* through the acetabulum shows a lucent nidus, which is partially calcified *(arrow)*. This is characteristic for an osteoid osteoma; however, osteomyelitis with a sequestrum could have an identical appearance except for the bone scan double density sign.

FIGURE 8-16 **Osteopathia striata.** Multiple linear dense streaks are seen in the distal femur, which are characteristic of osteopathia striata.

FIGURE 8-18 **Pachydermoperiostosis.** An anteroposterior film of the knee in this 50-year-old black man shows extensive periostitis about the knee, which is characteristic for pachydermoperiostosis.

drawing a line along the lateral femoral neck and noting that in normal subjects this line intersects about a quarter of the epiphysis (Fig. 8-20). In patients with a slipped capital epiphysis, this line intersects little or none of the slipped epiphysis. This process is often found bilaterally and is treated by internally fixing the epiphysis with pins.

FIGURE 8-17 **Osteopoikilosis.** An anteroposterior view of the pelvis reveals multiple small round sclerotic foci throughout the pelvis and femurs. This is diagnostic of osteopoikilosis. Metastatic disease is occasionally mistaken for this disorder.

FIGURE 8-19 **Sarcoid.** An anteroposterior plain film of the hands in a patient with sarcoidosis shows multiple lytic lesions, many of which demonstrate a "lacelike" pattern.

FIGURE 8-20 Slipped capital femoral epiphysis. A plain film of the hips in this child shows medial slippage of the left femoral capital epiphysis (*B*) as compared with the right (*A*). Although the amount of slippage is slight and difficult to appreciate at first glance, note that a line drawn along the lateral femoral neck on the normal side (*A*) intersects a portion of the femoral epiphysis, whereas on the left side (*B*) a similar line misses most of the epiphysis. A schematic of the normal hip and a hip with a slipped capital epiphysis (*C*) shows how a line parallel to the femoral neck (*solid line*) that is then moved to the lateral aspect of the femoral neck (*dotted line*) intersects part of the epiphysis (*shaded*) in the normal and misses the epiphysis in a slipped epiphysis.

REFERENCES

1. Mankin H: Nontraumatic necrosis of bone (osteonecrosis). N Engl J Med 1992;326:1473-1479.
2. Mitchell D, Kressel H, Arger P, et al: Avascular necrosis of the femoral head: Morphologic assessment by MR imaging, with CT correlation. Radiology 1986; 161:739-742.
3. Marcove R, Heelan R, Huvos A, et al: Osteoid osteoma. Diagnosis, localization, and treatment. Clin Orthop Relat Res 1991;267:197-201.
4. Helms CA, Hattner RS, Vogler J III: Osteoid osteoma: Radionuclide diagnosis. Radiology 1984;151(3): 779-784.

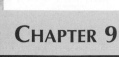

CHAPTER 9

Magnetic Resonance Imaging of the Knee

Magnetic resonance imaging (MRI) of the knee has developed into one of the most frequently requested examinations in radiology. This is not just because many people injure their knees, but because of its high accuracy in depicting internal derangements. Accuracy reports of knee MRI vary from 85 to 95% with many investigators believing that MRI of the knee is, in fact, more accurate than arthroscopy. Few top orthopedic surgeons will operate on a knee without an MRI to serve as a "road map." Although some surgeons feel MRI is too expensive for routine use in every patient, there are studies that show enormous financial savings (not to mention decreased patient morbidity) in performing an MR examination on every patient who is a candidate for knee arthroscopy. Many of these patients do not need subsequent arthroscopy and those who do benefit from a more complete preoperative assessment (not directly reflected in financial savings but clearly beneficial for surgical planning).[1] MRI of the knee has a high negative predictive value; therefore, a normal MRI knee examination is highly accurate in excluding an internal derangement.[2,3]

Maximum diagnostic accuracy can be obtained in several ways. First, and most obvious, is to obtain high-quality images. This includes using the appropriate imaging protocol. Using an inappropriate protocol is probably the number one error committed in knee MRI. Second, knowing the basic MRI signs for internal derangements is key in achieving a high accuracy rate. Third, knowing the imaging pitfalls, such as normal variants that can mimic pathology, will further aid in diagnostic accuracy. Proper protocols, basic imaging signs, and pitfalls are discussed in detail in this chapter.

IMAGING PROTOCOL

The proper imaging protocol is essential for a high diagnostic accuracy rate. A sagittal T1-weighted (or proton density) sequence is essential for examining the menisci. Slices of 4 or 5 mm in thickness with a small (12 to 14 cm) field of view and at least a 192 matrix are recommended. The knee should be imaged using a dedicated knee coil and externally rotated about 5 to 10 degrees (do not exceed 10 degrees) to put the anterior cruciate ligament (ACL) in the plane of imaging. T2 spin-echo or T2* gradient-echo sagittal images are obtained primarily to examine the cruciate ligaments and cartilage. With T2 spin-echo images, meniscal tears may be difficult to see; however, they will be picked up on the proton density images. Thus, the menisci and the cruciate ligaments are examined primarily on the sagittal images. Although the menisci and the cruciate ligaments can be seen on the coronal and axial images, it is rare for those images to show an abnormality that is not seen on the sagittal images.

Coronal images are obtained to examine the collateral ligaments and to look for meniscocapsular separations. These abnormalities can most often only be seen with T2-weighted images. T1 coronal images, therefore, are a waste of time, because there is nothing to be seen on these images that cannot be equally well seen on the sagittal images. T2* gradient-echo coronal or fast spin-echo (FSE) T2 sequences in the coronal plane are imperative. FSE (also called turbo spin-echo, or TSE) sequences should have fat suppression applied or fluid cannot be distinguished from fat.

A few centers continue to use T1-weighted coronal images without realizing that they give no additional information and, in fact, can hide significant abnormalities. Why would they do this? T1-weighted coronal images were part of everyone's protocol when we first began to use MRI in the knee. Articles, book chapters, and speakers (including me) would give the standard protocol, not thinking enough about what each sequence was showing us. I remember reading a knee study in the late 1980s with one radiology resident, and I asked him to hedge on the diagnosis of a partial tear of the medial collateral ligament (MCL) and request a repeat examination with T2-weighted coronals to rule out a meniscocapsular separation. This was the second or third time that week that the resident had been so instructed, so he asked, "Why don't we just routinely do a T2 coronal? We don't see anything on the T1 coronal, and we often have to hedge or repeat the exam with a T2 coronal." I just said for him to worry about dictating the cases, whereas I and others would take care of setting up the protocols. Well, 2 weeks later he rotated to another service, and we began doing T2 coronal images as part of our standard knee protocol. Uppity residents!

Axial images were initially used by the technologists as a scout view. They were then found to be useful for viewing the patellofemoral cartilage and for examining a medial patellar plica. As in the coronal images, to afford an opportunity to see any pathology, T2 or T2* images must be obtained.

We have found that fat suppressing the sagittal T1 or proton density meniscus-sensitive sequence increases the dynamic range of signal in the meniscus and makes meniscal pathology more conspicuous. It eliminates the distracting high signal in the marrow, making it easier to visualize the meniscus.

The use of FSE sequences with a short echo time (FSE proton density) has been shown in several reports to be useful for meniscal tears and in others to decrease sensitivity. What is the truth? The truth is that every published report I can find shows a sensitivity of around 80% for FSE proton density sequences, whereas conventional spin echo sequences have a sensitivity closer to 95%. It is very controversial, but basically everyone's results are the same (80% sensitivity), only the conclusions differ.[4] If you're willing to decrease your sensitivity for meniscal tears from 95 to 80% to save 3 minutes (the only advantage of FSE), then your time is more valuable than your diagnostic accuracy. Get another job!

The protocol I currently recommend consists of a sagittal proton-density weighted spin-echo series with fat suppression and sagittal, coronal, and axial FSE T2 with fat suppression (Table 9-1). Many acceptable variations of this protocol exist. Many centers, for various reasons, prefer not to use FSE images and instead use gradient-echo series.

MENISCI

The normal meniscus is a fibrocartilaginous, C-shaped structure that is uniformly low in signal on both T1- and T2-weighted sequences (Fig. 9-1). With T2* sequences the menisci will usually demonstrate some internal signal. With T1-weighted images any signal within the meniscus is abnormal, except in children, in whom some signal is normal and represents normal vascularity. Meniscal signal that does not disrupt an articular surface is representative of intrasubstance degeneration (Fig. 9-2), which is myxoid degeneration of the fibrocartilage. It most likely represents aging and normal wear and tear. It is not believed to be symptomatic and cannot be diagnosed clinically or with arthroscopy. Some choose, therefore, not to mention intrasubstance degeneration in the radiology interpretation. A grading scale for meniscal signal that is widely used is the following (Fig. 9-3): grade 1—rounded or amorphous signal that does *not* disrupt an articular surface; grade 2—linear signal that does *not* disrupt an articular surface; and grade 3—rounded or linear signal that disrupts an articular surface (Fig. 9-4). Grades 1 and 2 are intrasubstance degeneration and should not be reported as "grade 1 or 2 tears." This is a radiology grading scale that is not known widely by orthopedic surgeons; hence, the term *tear* often leads to an unnecessary arthroscopy (arthroscopy is not indicated for intrasubstance degeneration). Only grade 3 is a meniscal tear.

When high signal in a meniscus disrupts the superior or inferior articular surface, a meniscal tear is diagnosed (see Fig. 9-4). Care must be taken to be sure that the signal actually disrupts the articular surface of the meniscus before calling a tear. When high signal approaches the articular surface of the meniscus, it seems that many radiologists tend to overcall it regardless of whether it disrupts the surface. This is evidenced not only from my experience of watching residents and fellows but

TABLE 9-1   Knee Protocol

	TR/TE	Nex, n	Matrix	Fat suppression	Thickness, mm	FOV
Sagittal	2000/20	1	192	Yes	4	14
Sagittal	4000/70	2	192	Yes	4	14
Coronal	4000/70	2	192	Yes	4	14
Axial	4000/70	2	192	Yes	4	14

FOV, field of view; Nex, number of excitations; TE, echo time; TR, repetition time.

A

B

FIGURE 9-1 Normal meniscus. *A,* A T1-weighted sagittal image (TR, 600; TE, 30) through a normal lateral meniscus demonstrates uniform low signal in the meniscus. This is a section through the body of the meniscus, because it has a bowtie configuration. Two sections of the body should be seen in each meniscus with 4- or 5-mm-thick slices. *B,* In the same T1-weighted sequence, this sagittal image demonstrates uniform low signal in the anterior and posterior horns of this normal lateral meniscus. (Anterior is to the left.)

also from noting that most published series on accuracy of knee MRI have a lower specificity than sensitivity (i.e., there are more false-positives than false-negatives). One way to avoid false-positive calls is to cover up the meniscus with a card, or your thumbnail, leaving only a thin margin of the articular surface of the meniscus visible. If this margin of articular surface of the meniscus is seen as a straight uninterrupted line, no tear of the meniscus is present. If the thin margin is interrupted, a meniscal tear is present.

Meniscal tears have many different configurations and locations, with an oblique tear extending

A

B

FIGURE 9-2 Intrasubstance degeneration. *A,* Faint intermediate signal can be seen in the posterior horn of this meniscus *(arrow),* which does not disrupt the articular surface of the meniscus. This is intrasubstance degeneration. *B,* Linear high signal is present in the posterior body segment of the meniscus *(arrow).* The signal does not disrupt the articular surface; therefore, this represents intrasubstance degeneration.

GRADE 1   GRADE 2   GRADE 3

FIGURE 9-3 Grading scale for menisci. A schematic of the magnetic resonance imaging grading scale for meniscal abnormalities: grade 1 has rounded or amorphous signal in the meniscus that does not disrupt an articular surface. Grade 2 has linear signal that does not disrupt an articular surface. Grades 1 and 2 represent intrasubstance degeneration. Grade 3 has signal that disrupt an articular surface and indicates a meniscal tear.

to the inferior surface of the posterior horn of the medial meniscus the most common type. In a small but significant percentage of cases (around 10%), it can be virtually impossible to be certain if meniscal high signal disrupts an articular surface. In these cases, it is recommended that the surgeon be advised that it is too close to call. The surgeon can then rely on his clinical expertise to

FIGURE 9-4 Meniscal tear. This fat-suppressed T1-weighted sagittal image (TR, 600; TE, 30) shows linear high signal in the posterior horn of the meniscus, which disrupts the inferior articular surface. This is the appearance of an oblique meniscal tear.

decide if arthroscopy is warranted, and, if it is, the MRI will guide him to where the questionable tear is located. De Smet[5] showed that signal that disrupts the surface of the meniscus on only one sagittal image should be considered a sign of an equivocal tear. He found only 56% of the medial menisci and 30% of the lateral menisci were torn if only one sagittal image showed the "tear." If these equivocal cases are excluded, the remaining cases will have an extremely high accuracy rate.

Another common meniscus tear, one that is frequently missed by radiologists, is a bucket handle tear. This is a vertical longitudinal tear that can result in the inner free edge of the meniscus becoming displaced into the intercondylar notch (Fig. 9-5). It is most easily recognized by observing on the sagittal images that only one image is present that has the bowtie appearance of the body segment of the meniscus (Fig. 9-6). Normally, two

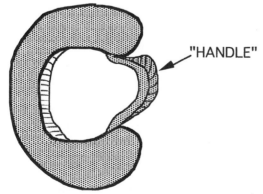

FIGURE 9-5 Bucket handle tear. This drawing illustrates a bucket handle tear with the torn free edge of the meniscus displaced as the "handle" of the bucket.

A

B

FIGURE 9-6 Bucket handle tear. Sagittal gradient-echo images through the medial meniscus at its most medial aspect reveal one bowtie, indicative of the body of the meniscus (A) with the adjacent image (B) having apparent normal anterior and posterior horns. However, because there should be two consecutive sagittal images with a bowtie configuration, this indicates a bucket handle tear. (Anterior is to the left.)

contiguous sagittal images with a bowtie shape are seen, because the normal meniscus is 9 to 12 mm in width and the sagittal images are 4 to 5 mm in thickness. On the coronal images a bucket handle tear may reveal the meniscus to be shortened and truncated; however, often, the torn meniscus remodels and truncation cannot be appreciated (Fig. 9-7). The displaced inner edge of the meniscus (the "handle" of the bucket) is often seen in the intercondylar notch on sagittal or coronal views (Fig. 9-8).

Another meniscus tear that is diagnosed by having too few bowtie segments present in the sagittal plane is a radial tear or parrot beak tear. This is a tear of the free edge of the meniscus (Fig. 9-9), which is a common tear but only occasionally causes enough symptoms by itself to warrant arthroscopy. It should be suspected when only one bowtie segment is present and the adjacent sagittal image shows a small gap (a bucket handle tear will have a large gap) in the expected bowtie (Fig. 9-10).

FIGURE 9-7 **Schematic of bucket handle tear.** This drawing shows how a vertical longitudinal tear as shown on the axial view *(left)* can appear on the coronal views *(right)*. Before the free edge is displaced the tear may be seen *(top right)*; after the free edge (or "handle") displaces the remaining meniscus may appear truncated *(center right)*; after weight bearing the truncated meniscus smooths out to a sharp triangle that is simply decreased in width from the normal *(bottom right)*.

FIGURE 9-8 **Displaced fragment in bucket handle tear.** A sagittal T1-weighted image through the intercondylar notch in a patient with a bucket handle tear reveals the displaced free fragment or "handle" *(arrows)* just anterior to the posterior cruciate ligament.

FIGURE 9-9 **Parrot beak tear.** This drawing shows the appearance of a radial free edge meniscal tear called a parrot beak tear.

FIGURE 9-10 **Radial tear.** Sagittal images through the body of the medial meniscus in a patient with a radial tear showed a normal bowtie configuration in the most medial image, with the next adjacent image (shown here) having a small gap *(arrow)*, which indicates a disruption of the free edge of the meniscus. Note the rounded tip of the apparent anterior horn, which is further evidence of a torn free edge or parrot beak tear.

The apparent anterior or posterior horn triangles, or both, will often be rounded or truncated instead of pointed.

Use of the "bowtie sign," that is, having two consecutive sagittal images that demonstrate a bowtie configuration, is one of the most useful signs I can give beginners in evaluating a knee MR image.[6] It will allow a bucket handle tear to virtually never be overlooked and, as the next section describes, can be used to diagnose a discoid meniscus. There are four pitfalls to be aware of in applying the bowtie sign (Table 9-2). First, if the knee and the menisci are small, as in a child's knee, only one bowtie may be observed without a bucket handle tear being present. However, there will be only two or three sagittal images that demonstrate the anterior and posterior horns. A normal-size knee will have two bowties and three or four images that show the anterior and posterior horns. Also, in a small knee, both the medial and lateral menisci will have only one bowtie image, and bucket han-

TABLE 9-2   Pitfalls in "Bowtie" Sign

1. Small knee with small menisci
2. Older patients (>60 years) who may have fraying and degeneration of free edge
3. Incomplete coverage
4. Prior surgery

dle tears involving both the medial and lateral menisci are rare.

The second pitfall in the bowtie sign is seen in patients older than 60 years. This is not a common age to have an internal derangement of the knee, but it does happen. Patients older than 60 years often have worn down the inner free edges of their menisci so that they only have one sagittal image of the body seen, followed by four or five images that show the anterior and posterior horns—usually a good sign for a bucket handle tear. This, unlike the pitfall described in children or small knees, does not necessarily occur in both menisci. How do I differentiate this from a real bucket handle tear? First, degenerative joint disease is always present, and, second, no displaced meniscal fragment can be found.

A third pitfall to be aware of in using the bowtie sign is that the sign only works if the entire meniscus is covered with sagittal images. If the technologist doesn't begin the sagittal images at the far medial or lateral aspects of the knee, the meniscus will not be imaged in its entirety. One will quickly learn to appreciate whether the entire meniscus is covered.

A discoid meniscus is a large disclike meniscus that can have many different shapes—lens shaped, wedged, flat, and others. It is not known if it is congenital or acquired, but most are found in children or young adults. It is seen laterally in up to 3% of the population, with a discoid medial meniscus being much less common. A discoid meniscus is believed to be more prone to tear than a normal meniscus and can be symptomatic even without being torn. Although they are easily identified on coronal images by noting meniscal tissue extending into the tibial spines at the intercondylar notch (Fig. 9-11), they are most reliably diagnosed by noting more than two consecutive sagittal images that show the meniscus with a bowtie appearance (Fig. 9-12). Hence, the bowtie sign can be used to

A

B

C

FIGURE 9-11 **Discoid lateral meniscus.** A coronal gradient-echo image through the intercondylar notch shows a large lateral meniscus with meniscal tissue extending into the notch medially (*arrow*).

FIGURE 9-12 **Discoid lateral meniscus.** Three consecutive 5-mm-thick T1-weighted images through the lateral meniscus, beginning with the most lateral (*A*) and extending medially (*B* and *C*); each show the meniscus to have a bowtie configuration. Because only two images should have a bowtie shape, indicative of the body of the meniscus, this is diagnostic of a discoid lateral meniscus (Fig. 9-11 is a coronal image of the same knee). (Anterior is to the left.)

diagnose a bucket handle tear (fewer than two bowties) or a discoid meniscus (more than two bowties). If slices thinner than 4 or 5 mm are used, the bowtie sign can be adjusted to whatever slice thickness is used.

The lateral meniscus often has what appears to be a tear on the anterior horn near its upper margin, which is a pseudotear from the insertion of the transverse ligament (Fig. 9-13). This can easily be differentiated from a real tear by following it medially across the knee in Hoffa's fat pad to where it inserts onto the anterior horn of the medial meniscus. Although less common than on the lateral meniscus, a pseudotear from the insertion of the transverse ligament onto the anterior horn of the medial meniscus can be seen.

Meniscal cysts occur in about 5% of cases and can cause pain even if the meniscus is not torn. The cause is unknown, but they occur more frequently in discoid menisci. If the meniscus is not torn, the surgical approach used by some is percutaneous with decompression and packing performed, whereas if a meniscus tear is associated with the cyst, it is approached intra-articularly. Hence, accurate diagnosis of a tear is imperative. The intrameniscal portion of the cyst typically does not get fluid-bright in signal on T2 sequences (Fig. 9-14), which has misled many radiologists into discounting the presence of a cyst. A meniscal cyst will enlarge the meniscus and give it a swollen appearance unless it decompresses into the soft tissues (called a parameniscal cyst) or into the joint through a meniscus tear. Decompression into a parameniscal cyst does not indicate a meniscus

A

B

FIGURE 9-14   **Meniscal cyst.** A sagittal proton density–weighted image (*A*) through the medial meniscus shows a swollen anterior horn filled with increased signal (*arrow*). A T2-weighted image (*B*) shows high signal similar to fluid in the parameniscal portion, whereas the intrameniscal signal is only intermediate.

FIGURE 9-13   **Pseudotear from a transverse ligament.** A sagittal T1-weighted image through the lateral meniscus shows linear high signal through the upper anterior horn (*arrow*), which resembles a tear. This is the insertion of the transverse ligament onto the meniscus (see Fig. 9-1*B* for another example). (Anterior is to the left.)

tear. A meniscus tear, by definition, has to disrupt the articular surface of the meniscus.

CRUCIATE LIGAMENTS

MRI of the cruciate ligaments is more accurate than MRI of the menisci, with accuracy reported near 100% in several published series.[7,8] The normal ACL is seen in the intercondylar notch as a linear, predominantly low-signal structure on T1- or proton density–weighted images that often shows some linear striations near its insertion onto the medial tibial spine when viewed on sagittal images (Fig. 9-15A). T2 or T2* images are imperative for obtaining the greatest accuracy in diagnosing ACL tears, because fluid and hemorrhage will often obscure the ligament on T1-weighted images (see Fig. 9-15B).

A torn ACL is most often simply not visualized (Fig. 9-16), although sometimes the actual disruption will be seen (Fig. 9-17). Partial tears or sprains of the ACL are manifested by high signal within an otherwise intact ligament. The diagnosis of a partial tear or sprain is generally not critical on MRI, because the treatment afforded the patient depends solely on the diagnosis of a complete tear. In most instances, a partial tear cannot be distinguished from an intact ACL at surgery.

An entity that is frequently mistaken for a torn ACL is an ACL cyst (Fig. 9-18). The cause is unknown, but it basically represents fluid in and around the fibers of the ACL, giving it a swollen, "drumstick" appearance on sagittal images. It has been mistakenly diagnosed as a tumor with subsequent radical removal (oops!) in one published report. It is an incidental finding with little or no clinical significance. It is found in about 1% of all knees. Although it often gets misdiagnosed as an ACL tear on MRI, it virtually never confuses a surgeon into operating, because the knee is stable.

The normal posterior cruciate ligament (PCL) is a gently curved, uniformly low-signal structure (Fig. 9-19), which is infrequently torn and even less frequently repaired by surgeons. When torn, it typically has a thickened appearance with diffuse intermediate signal throughout (Fig. 9-20). Most orthopedic surgeons do not even inspect the PCL at arthroscopy and do not repair it when torn, because it rarely is a cause of instability. A former fellow that I worked with tried to publish an MRI sign for a torn PCL. After collecting a dozen cases with torn posterior cruciates, he got the operative reports from the patients' records. We were surprised to find that not one surgeon even mentioned the PCL in any of the cases! We called a few of the surgeons and each gave the same answer— they virtually never repair the PCL, because it does not lead to instability; hence, they don't even bother to look at it during arthroscopy. Although not all surgeons ascribe to this philosophy, many do. If your surgeon does, it's a kind of freedom you have in looking at the posterior cruciate. You can tell them it's tied in a knot and it won't matter.

A low-signal round structure is often seen just anterior or posterior to the PCL on the sagittal views. A loose body or a free fragment of a piece of torn meniscus can have this appearance (Fig. 9-21),

A   **B**

Figure 9-15   **Normal anterior cruciate ligament (ACL).** *A,* A sagittal T1-weighted image through the intercondylar notch shows the normal appearance of the ACL *(arrows)*. *B,* A sagittal T2-weighted image with fat suppression through the intercondylar notch in another patient shows a normal ACL.

FIGURE 9-16 **Torn anterior cruciate ligament (ACL).** This sagittal T2-weighted image with fat suppression through the intercondylar notch fails to show the ACL. This is a fairly typical example of a completely torn ACL.

FIGURE 9-18 **Anterior cruciate ligament (ACL) cyst.** This sagittal T2-weighted image with fat suppression through the intercondylar notch shows the ACL with a drumstick appearance and high signal within. This is the appearance of an ACL cyst.

FIGURE 9-17 **Torn anterior cruciate ligament (ACL).** *A,* A sagittal gradient-echo image through the intercondylar notch shows fibers of a torn ACL, which are disrupted centrally *(arrow).*

FIGURE 9-19 **Normal posterior cruciate ligament (PCL).** A sagittal T1-weighted image through the intercondylar notch shows the appearance of the normal PCL with its characteristic uniform low signal *(arrow).*

FIGURE 9-20 **Torn posterior cruciate ligament (PCL).** A sagittal T1-weighted image through the intercondylar notch reveals the PCL to have a fat or thickened appearance with diffuse intermediate signal throughout. This is typical for a torn PCL.

FIGURE 9-21 **Free fragment of a torn meniscus.** A sagittal T1-weighted image through the intercondylar notch in this patient with a torn meniscus shows two rounded low-signal structures (*arrows*), which are free fragments of meniscal tissue. A meniscofemoral ligament of Wrisberg could have the appearance of either of these loose bodies.

but it is most commonly caused by a meniscofemoral ligament, which extends obliquely across the knee from the medial femoral condyle to the posterior horn of the lateral meniscus (Fig. 9-22). If it passes in front of the PCL, it is called the ligament of Humphry, and if it passes behind the PCL, it is the ligament of Wrisberg (Fig. 9-23). One or the other is present in up to 72% of all knees on MRI. In less than 5% of cases, both will be present.

The insertion of the ligament of Humphry or Wrisberg onto the lateral meniscus can produce a pseudotear similar to that caused by the transverse ligament on the anterior horn of the lateral meniscus (Fig. 9-24). Before calling a tear on the upper aspect of the posterior horn of the lateral meniscus, care must be taken to look for a meniscofemoral ligament to be certain it is not a pseudotear from the ligament's insertion. Similarly, before calling a loose body in front of or behind the PCL, care must be taken to try and follow the structure across to the lateral meniscus to determine if it is a meniscofemoral ligament.

COLLATERAL LIGAMENTS

The MCL originates on the medial femoral condyle and inserts on the tibia. It is closely applied to the joint and is intimately associated

FIGURE 9-22 **Ligament of Wrisberg.** This coronal T1-weighted image shows an obliquely oriented structure extending from the medial femoral condyle to the lateral meniscus. This is a normal ligament of Wrisberg.

with the medial joint capsule and the medial meniscus. The MCL is uniformly low in signal on all imaging sequences. Injuries to the MCL usually occur from a valgus stress, a blow to the lateral part of the knee. A grade 1 injury represents a mild

A

B

FIGURE 9-23 **Ligament of Wrisberg.** *A,* A sagittal T1-weighted image through the intercondylar notch shows a rounded low-signal structure posterior to the posterior cruciate ligament, which is the meniscofemoral ligament of Wrisberg *(arrow). B,* This drawing shows the relationship of the ligaments of Wrisberg and Humphry to the posterior cruciate ligament.

sprain and is diagnosed on MRI by noting fluid or hemorrhage in the soft tissues medial to the MCL (Fig. 9-25). The ligament is otherwise normal. A grade 2 injury is a partial tear and is seen as high signal in and around the MCL on T2 or T2* coronal sequences. The ligament is intact, although the deep or superficial fibers may show minimal disruption. A grade 3 injury is a complete disruption of the MCL. It can be best appreciated on T2 or T2* images (Fig. 9-26). It is unusual for a surgeon to operate on an MCL even if it is a complete disruption. MCL partial tears, and even complete tears, heal nicely with immobilization.

A meniscocapsular separation occurs when the medial meniscus is torn from its attachment to the

joint capsule. It occurs most commonly at the site of the MCL and often occurs concomitantly with an MCL injury. It is easily recognized on a T2 or T2* coronal image by noting joint fluid extending between the medial meniscus and the capsule. It is essential to use T2 or T2* sequences, because a T1-weighted image may not detect the fluid between the meniscus and the capsule (Fig. 9-27). They can be overlooked at arthroscopy if they involve only the superficial fibers of the capsule, because they are then essentially extracapsular. It is an important diagnosis to make, because it involves a vascular portion of the meniscus; hence, it will readily heal with immobilization or with suturing by the surgeon. If overlooked and continued activity occurs, it can lose the vascular interface and never heal.

The lateral collateral ligament consists of three parts. The most posterior structure is the tendon of the biceps femoris, which inserts onto the head of the fibula. Next, anterior to the biceps, is the true lateral collateral ligament, also called the fibulocollateral ligament, which extends from the lateral femoral condyle to the head of the fibula (Fig. 9-28). The biceps and the fibulocollateral ligament usually join and insert onto the head of the fibula in a conjoined manner. Anterior to the fibulocollateral ligament is the iliotibial band, which extends into the fascia more anteriorly and blends into the lateral retinaculum on the patella. The lateral collateral ligament complex is infrequently torn, but it can have significant long-term consequences of pain and instability in athletes if not treated aggressively. This is called posterolateral corner instability.

The posterolateral corner is basically the soft tissues in and around the lateral collateral ligament complex. These structures are injured in hyperextension and about 95% of the time are associated with a PCL or an ACL tear, or both.[9] If an ACL and/or PCL tear is present with a tear of two or more of the following structures—fibulocollateral ligament, biceps tendon, iliotibial band, popliteofibular ligament, popliteus tendon, and arcuate ligament—posterolateral corner instability should be suggested (Fig. 9-29). Some of the structures listed are hard to identify and take a lot of experience; therefore, one can simply suggest posterolateral corner injury if an ACL or PCL is torn and part of the lateral collateral ligament complex has a definite tear. This is a significant injury, and usually the surgeon appreciates a phone call, because many surgeons believe the posterolateral corner must be repaired promptly.

PATELLA AND CARTILAGE

The patellar cartilage commonly undergoes degeneration causing exquisite pain and tenderness.

FIGURE 9-24 **Pseudotear from ligament of Humphry insertion.** *A,* A sagittal, gradient-echo image through the lateral meniscus reveals an apparent tear of the posterior horn *(arrow).* *B,* On the adjacent image 3 mm more medially, the "tear" seems to widen *(arrow)* as the meniscus becomes less well seen. *C,* On the next adjacent image medially, a ligament of Humphry *(arrow)* is seen anterior to the posterior cruciate ligament. Note that the ligament of Humphry is a continuation of the structure seen on the prior image and extends into the upper part of the posterior horn of the lateral meniscus in *A.*

This is called chondromalacia patella. It can be diagnosed on sagittal images but is generally more reliably identified on axial images. Because hyaline articular cartilage has the same signal intensity as joint fluid on T1-weighted sequences, T2 or T2* sequences are necessary to diagnose chondromalacia patella.

Chondromalacia begins with focal swelling and degeneration of the cartilage. This can be seen as low- or high-signal foci in the cartilage. As it pro-

gresses, it causes thinning and irregularity of the articular surface of the cartilage, and finally underlying bone is exposed (Fig. 9-30).

A normal structure that is seen in more than half the population is the medial patellar plica. It is an embryologic remnant from when the knee was divided into three compartments. It is a thin fibrous band that extends from the medial capsule toward, and sometimes onto, the medial facet of the patella (Fig. 9-31). A suprapatellar and

FIGURE 9-25 **Grade 1 sprain of the medial collateral ligament (MCL).** A gradient-echo coronal image reveals high signal in the soft tissues adjacent to the MCL *(arrows)*, which represents edema and hemorrhage from a sprain of the MCL. The MCL is clearly intact; hence, a complete tear is easily excluded.

infrapatellar plica can also be present. The medial patellar plica can on rare occasions thicken and cause clinical symptoms indistinguishable from a torn meniscus, which has been termed plica syndrome (Fig. 9-32). T2 or T2* images are necessary to visualize a plica in most instances. An abnormal plica can be easily removed arthroscopically.

An abnormality that can clinically mimic plica syndrome, as well as mimic a torn meniscus, is bursitis. Two bursae typically are identified medially, which can become symptomatic. The first is the pes anserine bursa, which is somewhat uncommon. Three tendons, the sartorius, gracilis, and semitendinosus (remembered by the mnemonic "Some Girls Stand"), insert onto the anteromedial aspect of the tibia in a fan-shaped manner that has been likened to a goose's foot, hence the name pes anserinus. A bursa lies beneath the insertion site, which can become inflamed and cause medial joint line or patellar pain that can be confused with plica syndrome or a torn medial meniscus (Fig. 9-33). A second, much more common, medial bursa is the semimembranosus tibial collateral ligament bursa (an unwieldy name, to say the least!). It occurs at the medial joint line and often mimics a meniscal cyst. It has a characteristic comma shape as it drapes over the semimembranosus tendon (Fig. 9-34). Making the diagnosis of pes anserinus or semimembranosus tibial collateral ligament bursitis with MRI can prevent an unnecessary arthroscopy procedure—one in which the bursa would be overlooked, because they are extracapsular structures.

BONY ABNORMALITIES

The most frequently encountered bony abnormality seen with MRI is a contusion. A contusion

A **B**

FIGURE 9-26 **Torn medial collateral ligament (MCL).** *A,* A coronal gradient-echo image shows a large joint effusion with the MCL disrupted proximally *(arrow).* In addition, joint fluid can be seen extending between the medial meniscus and the MCL, which indicates a meniscocapsular separation. Neither of these diagnoses could be unequivocally made on the T1-weighted coronal image *(B).*

A   **B**

FIGURE 9-27   **Meniscocapsular separation.** *A,* A T1-weighted coronal image reveals a contusion of the lateral femoral condyle indicative of a valgus strain, which is often associated with a medial collateral ligament (MCL) tear. The MCL appears normal on this image; however, the linear low signal in the soft tissues just adjacent to the MCL is suggestive of fluid. This would indicate a partial tear or sprain of the MCL. *B,* A coronal gradient-echo image in the same knee reveals fluid between the medial meniscus and the MCL *(arrow),* which is diagnostic for a meniscocapsular separation. Faint high signal in the MCL and adjacent to it indicate a partial tear. A T2 or T2* sequence in the coronal plane are necessary to see these abnormalities.

FIGURE 9-28   **Normal lateral collateral ligament.** This coronal fast spin-echo T2 with fat suppression shows a normal fibulocollateral ligament (lateral collateral ligament) *(arrows)* extending from the lateral femoral condyle to the fibular head.

represents microfractures from trauma. They are also called bone bruises. They are easily identified on T1-weighted sequences as subarticular areas of inhomogeneous low signal (Fig. 9-35). With T2-weighting a contusion will show increased signal for several weeks, depending on its severity. It can be difficult to see increased signal with T2* images because of the susceptibility artifacts of the bone inherent with T2* images. Contusions can progress to osteochondritis dissecans if they are not treated with diminished weight bearing; hence, an isolated

bone contusion, with no other internal derangement, is a serious finding that requires treatment.

A commonly seen contusion is one that occurs on the posterior part of the lateral tibial plateau (Fig. 9-36). It is invariably associated with a torn ACL.[10] A kissing contusion on the lateral femoral condyle is often seen. When one or both of these contusions are present, an ACL tear is a virtual certainty. The only exception to this rule is in teenagers who are flexible enough to twist the knee and suffer the contusions while not tearing the ACL.

FIGURE 9-29   Posterolateral corner injury. *A,* This sagittal proton density image shows the posterior cruciate ligament (PCL) to be fat and increased in signal *(arrows),* indicative of a torn PCL. *B,* A coronal fast spin-echo (FSE) T2 with fat suppression reveals a tear of the lateral collateral ligament *(arrow). C,* An axial FSE T2 with fat suppression shows an injury to the popliteus tendon *(arrow)* with thickening and increased signal. This constellation of injuries indicates posterolateral corner instability.

FIGURE 9-30 **Chondromalacia patella.** An axial T2-weighted image through the patella in a patient who dislocated his patella shows a large chondral defect at the apex of the patella *(arrow)*. The hyaline articular cartilage was knocked off when the patella banged against the lateral femoral condyle during reduction.

FIGURE 9-32 **Thickened medial patellar plica.** This axial fast spin-echo T2-weighted image with fat suppression shows a thickened medial patellar plica *(arrow)*. This patient presented with a painful clicking knee, symptoms typical for either a torn meniscus or plica syndrome.

FIGURE 9-31 **Plica.** An axial gradient-echo image through the patella shows a low-signal linear structure *(arrow)* extending from the medial capsule toward the medial facet of the patella. This is a normal medial patellar plica. Without the joint effusion or the T2 weighting the plica would not be visualized.

FIGURE 9-33 **Pes anserinus bursitis.** A coronal T2* gradient-echo image shows a fluid collection below the medial joint line near the insertion of the pes anserinus tendons. This is pes anserinus bursitis.

A   **B**

FIGURE 9-34   **Semimembranosus tibial collateral ligament bursa.** *A,* A sagittal fast spin-echo (FSE) T2-weighted image with fat suppression through the medial aspect of the knee shows a fluid collection *(arrows)* at the joint line that is adjacent to the posterior horn of the medial meniscus. This is characteristic of a semimembranosus medial collateral ligament bursa. *B,* A coronal FSE T2-weighted image with fat suppression shows this bursa at the joint line with a comma-shaped appearance.

FIGURE 9-35   **Contusion.** A coronal fast spin-echo T2-weighted image with fat suppression shows a focus of high signal in the lateral femoral condyle, which is a characteristic appearance for a severe bone contusion. This occurred from a patella dislocation.

FIGURE 9-36   **Contusions.** A sagittal T1-weighted image through the lateral compartment shows irregular low signal in a subarticular location in the posterior tibial plateau and in the anterior part of the lateral femoral condyle. These findings are characteristic for bone contusions. This distribution of contusions in the posterior lateral tibial plateau and anterior in the lateral femoral condyle is almost always associated with a torn anterior cruciate ligament.

MRI is useful to examine fractures of the knee. Tibial plateau fractures can be imaged precisely with computed tomography; however, MRI allows soft tissues, internal derangements, and any bony abnormalities to be seen.

REFERENCES

1. Ruwe P, Wright J, Randall R, et al: Can MR imaging effectively replace diagnostic arthroscopy? Radiology 1992;183:335-339.
2. Crues JI, Mink J, Levy T, et al: Meniscal tears of the knee: Accuracy of MR imaging. Radiology 1987;164:445-448.
3. Mink JH, Deutsch AL: Magnetic resonance imaging of the knee. Clin Orthop Relat Res 1989;244:29-47.
4. Helms CA: The meniscus: Recent advances in MR imaging of the knee. AJR Am J Roentgenol 2002;179(5):1115-1122.
5. De Smet AA, Norris MA, Yandow DR, et al: MR diagnosis of meniscal tears of the knee: Importance of high signal in the meniscus that extends to the surface. AJR Am J Roentgenol 1993;161:101-107.
6. Helms CA, Laorr A, Cannon WD Jr: The absent bow tie sign in bucket-handle tears of the menisci in the knee. AJR Am J Roentgenol 1998;170(1):57-61.
7. Lee J, Yao L, Phelps C, et al: Anterior cruciate ligament tears: MR imaging compared with arthroscopy and clinical tests. Radiology 1988;166:861-864.
8. Mink J, Levy T, Crues JI: Tears of the anterior cruciate ligament and menisci of the knee: MR imaging evaluation. Radiology 1988;167:769-774.
9. Covey DC: Injuries of the posterolateral corner of the knee. J Bone Joint Surg Am 2001;83-A:106-118.
10. Murphy B, Smith R, Uribe J, et al: Bone signal abnormalities in the posterolateral tibia and lateral femoral condyle in complete tears of the anterior cruciate ligament: A specific sign? Radiology 1992;182:221-224.

CHAPTER 10

Magnetic Resonance Imaging of the Shoulder

Magnetic resonance imaging (MRI) of the shoulder is one of the more difficult examinations to interpret that I see on a regular basis. It has been shown to have a high degree of accuracy, especially when performed with arthrography.[1,2] Although most texts divide the shoulder into either cuff or labral abnormalities, it is important to know that cuff and labral pathology often coexist, causing great confusion in the clinical presentation and the physical examination. Most surgeons are aware that failure to address a labral abnormality when fixing a torn cuff can result in unsuccessful surgical results, and, conversely, fixing a labral abnormality and ignoring a cuff problem may not address the patient's real problem. MRI can show both the cuff and the labrum to good advantage. Also, MRI of the shoulder may reveal one of the entities I will discuss in the last part of this chapter, such as suprascapular nerve entrapment, quadrilateral space syndrome, or Parsonage-Turner syndrome, any one of which can present similarly to a cuff problem.

ANATOMY

The rotator cuff is composed of the tendons of four muscles that converge on the greater and lesser tuberosities of the humerus: the supraspinatus, infraspinatus, subscapularis, and teres minor (Fig. 10-1). Of these, the supraspinatus is the one that most commonly causes clinically significant problems and is almost exclusively the one that is addressed surgically.

The supraspinatus tendon lies just superior to the scapula and inferior to the acromioclavicular (AC) joint and the acromion. It inserts into the greater tuberosity of the humerus. One to 2 cm proximal to its insertion is a section of the tendon called the "critical zone." This area is reported to have decreased vascularity and is therefore less

likely to heal after trauma. It is also the area of the tendon that undergoes fibrillar and myxoid degeneration (also called tendinopathy), presumably from aging and trauma, although this has not been proved. The critical zone of the supraspinatus tendon is where most rotator cuff tears occur, although a considerable number occur at the bone–tendon interface.

The glenoid labrum is a fibrocartilaginous ring that surrounds the periphery of the bony glenoid of the scapula. It serves as an attachment site for the capsule and broadens the base of the glenohumeral joint to allow increased stability. Tears of the glenoid labrum most commonly occur from, and result in, humeral head instability and dislocations.

IMAGING PROTOCOL

There are many variations in the imaging protocol that are all acceptable for showing normal and pathologic findings in the shoulder. The rotator cuff, that is, the supraspinatus tendon, is best seen on oblique coronal images that are aligned parallel to the supraspinatus muscle (Fig. 10-2). T2-weighted sequences, or acceptable variations, are mandatory. A commonly used protocol is a spin-echo proton density and T2-weighted sequence. Some prefer to use a spin-echo T1-weighted image in conjunction with a gradient echo or other type of T2* sequence. A more recent addition, as a substitute for more conventional T2-weighted images, is a fast spin-echo (FSE) T2 with fat suppression. The slice thickness should be no greater than 5 mm, and 3 mm is preferable. As with most joint imaging, a small field of view (16–20 cm) is recommended. A dedicated shoulder coil or a surface coil placed anteriorly over the shoulder is necessary, although no particular type of shoulder coil appears to be clearly superior.

FIGURE 10-1 Schematic of shoulder anatomy. This drawing shows the rotator cuff muscles in a sagittal plane (anterior is on the left). A, acromion; C, coracoid; H, humeral head.

FIGURE 10-2 Scout view for oblique coronal images. This axial image through the supraspinatus shows the cursors angled along the plane of the supraspinatus muscle (anterior on top). H, Humeral head.

The glenoid labrum is best seen on axial T2-weighted images. T1-weighted images do not give any additional information and can be eliminated. If a joint effusion is present, the labrum is easily identified. Without fluid in the joint it can be more difficult to clearly see the labrum; therefore, many radiologists will perform an MR arthrogram. Either saline alone or saline mixed with a small amount of gadolinium (a ratio of 1:200 is recommended) can be injected into the joint followed by MRI. MR arthrography is a routine part of shoulder imaging in many centers.

The oblique sagittal sequence is one of the most useful and is performed in our protocol as a standard T1-weighted sequence without fat suppression (to identify fatty atrophy) and as a FSE sion to identify fatty atrophy) and as a FSE T2-weighted sequence with fat suppression. This is useful in identifying cuff tears, fluid collections about the shoulder, and muscle edema. With T2 weighting, fluid in the subacromial bursa can occasionally be seen to better advantage than on the oblique coronal images. Also, this is the only sequence in which the shape of the acromion can be reliably identified, although it is not critical to note the shape of the acromion.

ROTATOR CUFF

The rotator cuff commonly suffers from what has been termed impingement syndrome. This was first described by Neer, an orthopedic surgeon, who claims that 95% of all rotator cuff tears occur from impingement syndrome. Impingement of the critical zone of the supraspinatus tendon occurs from abduction or flexion of the humerus, which allows the tendon to be impinged between the anterior acromion and the greater tuberosity. The tendon can also be impinged by the undersurface of the AC joint if downward pointing osteophytes or a thickened capsule are present. Other theories exist for impingement syndrome, including natural degeneration from aging and a predisposition for the critical zone to undergo degeneration because of decreased blood supply.[3] Most investigators agree that, whatever the cause, the natural course of impingement syndrome leads to a complete, or full-thickness, tear of the rotator cuff.

Treatment of impingement syndrome consists of rest, subacromial bursa steroid injections, and, if refractory to conservative care, surgery. Surgery involves removal of the anterior third of the acromion, resection of the coracoacromial ligament, and removal of any irregularities on the undersurface of the AC joint. If a tear of the supraspinatus tendon is present, it is repaired. Because the treatment for impingement syndrome is the same whether an actual cuff tear is present or not, the role of imaging in the diagnosis of cuff abnormalities has been questioned by some prominent surgeons.[4]

In examining the rotator cuff the anterior most oblique coronal images will show the critical zone of the supraspinatus tendon. A useful landmark for noting the supraspinatus tendon is the AC joint, which is an anterior structure and usually is easily located. The infraspinatus tendon is seen on the more posterior images and can easily be mistaken for the tendon of the supraspinatus. The supraspinatus tendon can be differentiated from the infraspinatus by noting the more horizontal course of the supraspinatus as compared with the infraspinatus, which runs obliquely inferiorly to superiorly.

The normal supraspinatus tendon is said to be uniformly low in signal on all pulse sequences. Unfortunately, this is not always the case. In fact, it usually has some intermediate to high signal in the critical zone (Fig. 10-3), which has caused much confusion in the evolution of interpreting shoulder MRI examinations. We imaged about 20 "normal" volunteers (residents and fellows) in the early days of learning shoulder MRI and only found 1 or 2 that had uniform low signal throughout the critical zone. This was very distressing because the literature at that time said any high signal in the critical zone meant it was abnormal. We know now that there are many causes for intermediate to high signal on T1-weighted images in the normal shoulder. We no longer even obtain an oblique coronal T1-weighted sequence because it does not add any additional information to the oblique coronal FSE T2-weighted sequence.

If signal in the critical zone is brighter on the T2-weighted images, it is abnormal and represents either tendonitis or a partial tear (severe tendonitis) (Fig. 10-4). However, if it disappears or has the same signal intensity as the adjacent muscle on T2-weighted sequences, it may represent one of many different processes:

1. Partial volume averaging of peritendinous fat can cause some high signal in the supraspinatus tendon on the oblique coronal images that does not get brighter on T2-weighted images.

2. If the plane of the oblique coronal images is slightly off of the plane of the tendon, muscle slips can be partially volume-averaged, which may appear as relatively high signal on T1-weighted images but will not get brighter with T2 images.

FIGURE 10-4 **Partial tear of the supraspinatus.** A T2-weighted oblique coronal image with fat saturation shows high signal in the critical zone of the supraspinatus tendon (*arrow*) with the tendon appearing very irregular. A small amount of fluid is seen in the subacromial bursa. Arthroscopy confirmed a partial tear on the bursal side of the supraspinatus tendon.

3. The so-called magic angle effect can cause apparent high signal in a tendon that lies at 55 degrees to the bore of the magnet (as does the critical zone of the supraspinatus tendon).[5] This high signal will not be seen on T2-weighted images (or any sequence with a long echo time). This is believed to be a common cause of high signal in the critical zone on T1-weighted images.

4. Myxoid or fibrillar degeneration of the supraspinatus tendon are commonly found in autopsy specimens, which increase with age. The majority of asymptomatic shoulders in patients older than 50 years are believed to have some tendon degeneration in the supraspinatus, which has been termed *tendinopathy*. This is seen as intermediate to high signal in the critical zone on T1-weighted images that does not increase with T2 weighting.[6] Similar to the myxoid degeneration that occurs in the menisci of the knee, it has not been shown that this is symptomatic.

5. Marked internal rotation of the humeral head can cause the infraspinatus tendon to lie superior to the supraspinatus tendon and cause an apparent "gap" in the supraspinatus tendon on the oblique coronal image when both tendons are seen on the same slice.[7] Care should be taken to study the

FIGURE 10-3 **Normal supraspinatus tendon.** A T1-weighted oblique coronal image in an asymptomatic man shows some increased signal in the critical zone of the supraspinatus tendon (*arrow*). As described in the text, there are many reasons why this can be found in the normal shoulder. It is imperative to note that the high signal does not increase on T2-weighted images.

patient with the arm in a neutral position or in external rotation.

6. Calcium deposits in the brain and lumbar spine discs have been described to occasionally cause high signal on T1-weighted images. Because calcification is often found in the critical zone of the supraspinatus tendon, it is reasonable to assume that these calcium deposits could occasionally be a source of intermediate to high signal on T1-weighted images. As in the brain and spine, the high signal on T1-weighted images would disappear or decrease on T2-weighted images.

Because high signal can be seen in the critical zone of the supraspinatus in a variety of normal situations, how can one differentiate the normal from the abnormal? So long as the T2-weighted images do not show the signal getting brighter, it probably does not matter. Tendon degeneration (tendinopathy) can be seen in asymptomatic shoulders of all ages; hence, it needs to be correlated with the clinical picture. If the signal gets brighter on T2-weighted images, it must be considered pathologic—either tendonitis or a partial tear. If, in addition, fluid is present in the subacromial bursa, a small full-thickness tear is a possibility even if a definite tendon disruption cannot be seen. A small amount of fluid can be seen in the subacromial bursa because of a partial tear.

If disruption of the supraspinatus tendon can be seen, obviously a full-thickness tear is present (Fig. 10-5). In these cases, fluid is invariably

A   **B**

C

FIGURE 10-5   **Torn supraspinatus (three examples).** *A,* An oblique coronal proton density image shows disruption of the supraspinatus tendon (*arrow*) and fluid in the subacromial bursa, which is seen surrounding the torn tendon. *B,* This oblique coronal fast spin-echo (FSE) T2-weighted image with fat suppression shows a gap in the supraspinatus tendon (*arrow*). *C,* This oblique coronal FSE T2-weighted image with fat suppression shows a gap in the supraspinatus tendon (*arrow*).

present in the subacromial bursa. Care should be taken to look for retraction of the supraspinatus muscle, because marked retraction will obviate some types of surgery.

I have found that three basic categories exist for the appearance of the supraspinatus tendon:

1. *Normal*—high signal on T1-weighted images that does not get brighter on T2-weighted images. This can represent one of several processes in a normal tendon or myxoid degeneration, also called tendinopathy. This should basically be considered "normal" because it has not been proven that tendinopathy is symptomatic.

2. *Tendonitis (or tendinosis)*—high signal on T1-weighted images that gets brighter on T2-weighted sequences. Little or no fluid is present in the subacromial bursa. This represents tendonitis or a partial tear.

3. *Cuff tear*—tendon disruption; a gap must be seen to call a full-thickness cuff tear.

It is generally easy to place the MRI appearance of the rotator cuff into one of these three categories, and a high degree of accuracy in diagnosing the state of the rotator cuff can be expected.

PARTIAL TEARS

Partial cuff tears have marked clinical significance because most agree that they will not heal on their own if they are greater than 25% of the cuff thickness.[8] Although we generally can't be so precise as to what percentage of the cuff is involved, we can usually identify partial cuff tears. If there is an irregularity or thinning of the cuff on either the bursal side of the cuff (see Fig. 10-4) or on the joint side, I will describe it as small, medium, or large (near full thickness).

A particular type of articular-sided partial tear has been described that is commonly seen. This has been termed a rim rent tear (Fig. 10-6). It occurs at the insertion of the fibers of the cuff onto the greater tuberosity. It most commonly occurs anteriorly at the insertion of the supraspinatus.

BONY ABNORMALITIES

The undersurface of the anterior acromion and the AC joint should be examined for osteophytes or irregularities that can be responsible for impingement syndrome (Fig. 10-7). In the proper clinical setting, an anterior acromioplasty will relieve the symptoms of impingement syndrome and prevent a more serious full-thickness cuff tear. It is imperative that the surgeon also remove any AC joint undersurface irregularity, if present, or unsuccessful surgical results can be expected.

A

B

FIGURE 10-6   **Rim rent tear.** *A,* This oblique coronal fast spin-echo (FSE) T2-weighted image with fat suppression shows linear increased signal at the insertion of the supraspinatus *(arrow)*. *B,* The oblique sagittal FSE T2-weighted image with fat suppression shows the same finding located anteriorly *(arrow)*. This is a partial tear on the articular side of the cuff.

The acromion has been classified into three types as seen on the sagittal images. The normal appearance, type 1, is an acromion with a flat or slightly convex undersurface; a type 2 acromion has a concave undersurface; and type 3 has a concave undersurface with an anterior osteophyte. Although it has been reported that a type 3

FIGURE 10-7 **Acromioclavicular (AC) joint osteophytes.** An oblique coronal T1-weighted image reveals osteophytes extending inferiorly off of the AC joint (*arrow*). This is a common source of impingement on the supraspinatus tendon.

FIGURE 10-8 **Os acromiale.** An axial fast spin-echo T2-weighted image with fat suppression through the upper part of the shoulder shows an unfused apophysis of the acromion, which is an os acromiale. The AC joint is seen anteriorly.

acromion is seen in up to 80% of cuff tears, type 2 is seen in 20%, and type 1 has no association with a torn cuff, this has not been substantiated, and it has certainly not been true in my experience. I frequently see cuff tears with a type 1 acromion, and I often see no cuff tear when a type 3 acromion is present. I do not routinely report the type of acromion because our surgeons don't use the information for anything. More importantly, I try to tell them if the acromion is low-lying or if it is anteriorly or laterally sloping, because it can cause bony impingement in these instances.

In about 5% of the population the distal acromion fails to fuse with the scapula leaving an unfused apophysis called an os acromiale (Fig. 10-8). The deltoid inserts on the acromion and, if a mobile os acromiale is present, it can pull the acromion down like a flap with resultant cuff impingement. Because the surgeon cannot see this at arthroscopy (or with open surgery), it is imperative to identify an os acromiale before surgery so the surgeon can consider fusing it.

Abnormalities of the humeral head include sclerosis and cystic changes about the greater tuberosity that are commonly present in patients with impingement syndrome and rotator cuff tears. Bony impaction on the posterosuperior aspect of the humeral head can be seen in patients with anterior instability of the humeral head. This is called a Hill-Sachs lesion and is best identified on the most superior two or three axial images (Fig. 10-9). The normal humeral head should be

FIGURE 10-9 **Hill-Sachs lesion.** An axial T1-weighted image through the superior portion of the humeral head shows a posterior impaction (*arrow*) caused by the glenoid labrum during an anterior dislocation of the humerus. This has been termed a Hill-Sachs lesion.

round on the superior slices—an irregularity posteriorly is abnormal.

GLENOID LABRUM

Tears or detachment of the glenoid labrum results in glenohumeral joint instability. They are commonly caused by dislocations, but less traumatic episodes, such as repeated trauma from throwing, can result in labral tears. Torn or detached labra are often repaired arthroscopically with good results. Labrum and rotator cuff abnormalities often coexist and an abnormality of one can lead to an abnormality in the other.

The normal labrum is a triangular-shaped, low-signal structure as viewed on an axial image, with the anterior labrum usually larger than the posterior labrum (Fig. 10-10). The anterior labrum is much more commonly involved with tears than the posterior, and the superior labrum is said to be rarely involved. In fact, the superior labrum, in my experience, is torn as often as the posterior labrum. The superior labrum is best evaluated on the oblique coronal views. Tears of the superior labrum are called SLAP lesions (superior labrum anterior to posterior). They are said to be seen mostly in throwing athletes as a result of the insertion of the long head of the biceps tendon onto the labrum avulsing part of the labrum during a forceful throwing motion.

If no joint effusion is present, a labral tear can be difficult to see unless it is extremely large. If joint fluid extends between the bony glenoid and the base of the labrum, a detached labrum is present. Tears in the body of the labrum are diagnosed by noting fluid extending into the labrum, by truncation of the labrum, or by fluid extending between the labrum and the bony glenoid (Fig. 10-11). The attachment of the glenohumeral ligaments to the labrum can cause a linear high signal that can mimic a tear (Fig. 10-12); therefore, care must be taken to be certain high-signal fluid is actually present in the tear.[9]

FIGURE 10-11 **Torn labrum.** An axial fast spin-echo T2-weighted image with fat suppression shows a tear of the anterior labrum *(arrow)*.

Several variations of normal exist in the labrum that can be confused for pathologic conditions. The most common one is seen in the superior labrum at the biceps attachment. This is a sublabral recess (Fig. 10-13), which can be difficult, at times, to differentiate from a SLAP tear. It should only be seen near the anterior portion of the superior labrum where the biceps attaches, and should

FIGURE 10-10 **Normal labrum.** An axial T2* gradient-echo image shows a normal anterior *(white arrow)* and posterior *(black arrow)* glenoid labrum. The anterior labrum is usually larger than the posterior.

FIGURE 10-12 **Insertion of glenohumeral ligament.** This axial T2* gradient-echo image reveals linear intermediate signal extending obliquely across the anterior labrum *(arrow)*, which simulates a tear. This is the insertion of the middle glenohumeral ligament onto the labrum.

A

FIGURE 10-13 **Sublabral recess.** A coronal T1-weighted gadolinium arthrogram with fat suppression shows fluid between the superior labrum and the cartilage of the bony glenoid, which is thin and smooth. This is a sublabral recess.

be thin and smooth in configuration. It is found in up to 40% of shoulders, and, quite frankly, I often find cases in which I cannot confidently tell if it is a sublabral recess or a SLAP tear.

Another commonly seen variant, found in 10 to 20% of shoulders, is a sublabral foramen. Like the sublabral recess, it has the appearance of a detached labrum (Fig. 10-14); however, it is differentiated from a detached labrum by its location in the anterosuperior quadrant of the glenoid—a location that is virtually immune from isolated labral pathology. A much less common variant is the Buford complex. It consists of an absent anterosuperior labrum with a thickened, cordlike middle glenohumeral ligament (Fig. 10-15). It is found in only about 1 to 3% of shoulders.

BICEPS TENDON

The long head of the biceps tendon runs in the bicipital groove between the greater and lesser tuberosities and inserts onto the superior labrum. It can be impinged by an abnormal acromion in the same way the supraspinatus tendon is impinged, resulting in tenosynovitis or tendonitis. In tenosynovitis, fluid can be seen in the tendon sheath surrounding an otherwise normal tendon. Because fluid in the glenohumeral joint can normally fill the biceps tendon sheath, this diagnosis is difficult to make with MRI alone. If the tendon is enlarged and/or has signal within it, tendonitis is present (Fig. 10-16). If the tendon is not seen on one or more of the axial images, it is disrupted (Fig. 10-17) or dislocated. Dislocation is uncom-

B

FIGURE 10-14 **Sublabral foramen.** *A,* An axial fast spin-echo T2-weighted image with fat suppression through the glenohumeral joint at the level of the coracoid shows a space between the anterior labrum and the bony glenoid *(white arrow),* which is a sublabral foramen. A detached labrum could have this appearance, but this is in the anterosuperior part of the joint. The middle glenohumeral ligament *(black arrow)* is seen as a separate structure anterior to the labrum. *B,* A few slices inferiorly the labrum is seen attached firmly to the anterior glenoid.

mon, but when it occurs, the tendon can be seen to lie anteromedial to the bicipital groove (Fig. 10-18).

SUPRASCAPULAR NERVE ENTRAPMENT

The suprascapular nerve is made up of branches from the C-4, C-5, and C-6 roots of the brachial plexus. It runs superior to the scapula, from anterior to posterior, just medial to the coracoid process. It gives off a branch that innervates the

FIGURE 10-15   Buford complex. *A,* An axial fast spin-echo T2-weighted image with fat suppression through the upper part of the joint shows the anterior labrum separated from the bony glenoid *(arrow)*. *B,* Lower in the joint the anterior labrum is firmly attached to the glenoid, but a thick, cordlike middle glenohumeral ligament is present *(arrow)*. This is a Buford complex. In *A* the anterior labrum is absent and a thick middle glenohumeral ligament is simulating the anterior labrum.

supraspinatus muscle as it courses posteriorly in the suprascapular notch. It then innervates the infraspinatus as it runs through the spinoglenoid notch in the posterior scapula. A not uncommon finding is a ganglion in the spinoglenoid notch that impresses the infraspinatus portion of the nerve with resultant pain and atrophy of the infraspinatus muscle (Fig. 10-19).[10] It has a near 100% association with a torn or detached posterior labrum. This has been reported almost exclusively in male individuals who are athletic, particularly weightlifters. It is important to see on preoperative MRI because the ganglion is extracapsular and cannot be seen at arthroscopy.

FIGURE 10-16   Biceps tendinitis. An axial gradient-echo image shows the biceps tendon *(arrow)* to be swollen and filled with high signal indicating tendonitis.

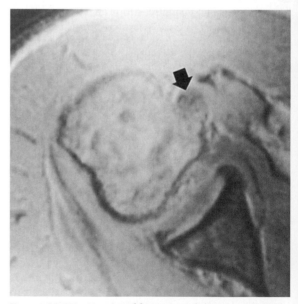

FIGURE 10-17   Ruptured biceps tendon. An axial gradient-echo image shows the biceps tendon sheath filled with fluid *(arrow)* but with no tendon. This indicates a torn biceps tendon.

FIGURE 10-18   **Dislocated biceps tendon.** This axial gradient-echo image shows an empty bicipital groove *(arrow)*, suggesting a torn biceps tendon; however, the biceps tendon is dislocated and can be seen anterior to the labrum *(curved arrow)*.

FIGURE 10-19   **Ganglion in spinoglenoid notch.** An axial T2 image reveals a high-signal mass posterior to the scapula in the spinoglenoid notch *(arrow)*. This is a ganglion that has impressed the suprascapular nerve causing shoulder pain and atrophy of the infraspinatus muscle.

FIGURE 10-20   **Quadrilateral space syndrome.** This oblique sagittal T1-weighted image shows fatty atrophy of the teres minor muscle *(arrow)*, which is diagnostic of quadrilateral space syndrome.

QUADRILATERAL SPACE SYNDROME

My search pattern for a shoulder MRI begins with the oblique sagittal T1-weighted images to look for fatty atrophy in any of the cuff muscles. If the infraspinatus is smaller than the other muscles and/or has fatty infiltration the aforementioned suprascapular nerve entrapment secondary to a ganglion in the spinoglenoid notch is the likely diagnosis. If the teres minor has fatty atrophy (Fig. 10-20), the only diagnosis I'm aware of is

quadrilateral space syndrome. This most commonly occurs from fibrous bands or scar tissue in the quadrilateral space impinging on the axillary nerve. The quadrilateral space lies between the teres minor superiorly, the teres major inferiorly, the long head of the triceps medially, and the diaphysis of the humerus laterally. The axillary nerve traverses the quadrilateral space and innervates the teres minor and deltoid muscles; however, the deltoid is rarely involved in quadrilateral space syndrome. We have found quadrilateral space syndrome in about 1% of our shoulder MRIs. These patients present with symptoms clinically similar to a rotator cuff tear, and I have seen several patients who have had needless surgery for presumed cuff pathology when the real problem was quadrilateral space syndrome. Generally, no surgery is necessary because physical therapy is usually successful in breaking up the fibrous bands or scar tissue that cause this entity.

PARSONAGE-TURNER SYNDROME

After I look at the oblique sagittal T1-weighted images for fatty atrophy I look at the oblique sagittal FSE T2-weighted fat suppressed images for muscle edema. In about 1% of cases neurogenic edema is found in muscle groups that correspond to a particular nerve (i.e., supraspinatus/infraspinatus = suprascapular nerve; teres minor/deltoid = axillary nerve). This is characteristic for Parsonage-Turner syndrome (Fig. 10-21). It's not pathognomonic because a traumatic nerve injury (such as a brachial plexus injury) could have a similar appearance. It becomes pathognomonic once the clinical presentation is provided. If there is no history of trauma or of an insidious onset and if the onset is sudden, with severe pain, followed in a day or two with profound weakness, the edema pattern is virtually pathognomonic for Parsonage-Turner syndrome.

FIGURE 10-21   **Parsonage-Turner syndrome.** An oblique sagittal T2-weighted image with fat suppression shows edema in the supraspinatus (S) and the infraspinatus (I) muscles consistent with involvement of the suprascapular nerve. The sudden onset with no history of trauma is characteristic for Parsonage-Turner syndrome.

The cause of Parsonage-Turner syndrome is unknown, but it seems to have an association with prior vaccinations, viral illness, or general anesthesia in about one third of cases. It is bilateral in about 10 to 15% of cases. It affects all ages of both sexes and is self-limited. It can affect either the axillary or suprascapular nerve, or both simultaneously. I have seen unnecessary shoulder, brachial plexus, and cervical spine surgery performed before the correct diagnosis of Parsonage-Turner syndrome was made.

Parsonage-Turner syndrome was first described in the radiology literature in 1998 indicating we all missed it on MRI for more than 15 years.[11] That's because we did not routinely fat suppress our shoulder images until the early 1990s, and the edema in the muscles was not conspicuous enough to be picked up on non–fat-suppressed sequences.

REFERENCES

1. Zlatkin MB, Iannotti JP, Roberts MC, et al: Rotator cuff tears: Diagnostic performance of MR imaging. Radiology 1989;172:223-229.
2. Palmer W, Brown J, et al: Rotator cuff: Evaluation with fat-suppressed MR arthrography. Radiology 1993;188:683-688.
3. Neviaser R, Neviaser T: Observations on impingement. Clin Orthop Relat Res 1990;254:60-63.
4. Rockwood C, Lyons F: Shoulder impingement syndrome: Diagnosis, radiographic evaluation, and treatment with a modified Neer acromioplasty. J Bone Joint Surg 1993;75-A:409-424.
5. Erickson S, Cox I, Hyde J, et al: Effect of tendon orientation on MR imaging signal intensity: A manifestation of the "magic angle" phenomenon. Radiology 1991;181:389-392.
6. Kjellin I, Ho CP, Cervilla V, et al: Alterations in the supraspinatus tendon at MR imaging: Correlation with histopathologic findings in cadavers. Radiology 1991;181:837-841.
7. Davis S, Teresi L, Bradley W, et al: Effect of arm rotation on MR imaging of the rotator cuff. Radiology 1991;181:265-268.
8. Fukuda H: The management of partial-thickness tears of the rotator cuff. J Bone Joint Surg Br 2003; 85:3-11.
9. Kaplan P, Bryans K, Davick J, et al: MR imaging of the normal shoulder: Variants and pitfalls. Radiology 1992;184:519-524.
10. Fritz R, Helms C, Steinbach L, Genant H: Suprascapular nerve entrapment: Evaluation with MR imaging. Radiology 1992;182:437-444.
11. Helms CA, Martinez S, Speer KP, et al: Acute brachial neuritis (Parsonage-Turner syndrome): MR imaging appearance—report of three cases. Radiology 1998; 207:255-259.

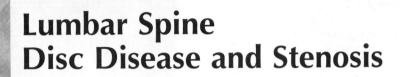

CHAPTER 11

Lumbar Spine
Disc Disease and Stenosis

Imaging the lumbar spine for disc disease and stenosis has evolved in the last 10 years from predominantly myelography-oriented examinations to plain computed tomography (CT) and magnetic resonance imaging (MRI) examinations. Multiple studies have shown that myelography, in addition to being invasive, is not as accurate as CT or MRI,[1-4] yet myelography continues to be performed. There is little justification for a lumbar myelogram for disc disease or stenosis in this era.

Although few differences between CT and MRI have been noted concerning diagnostic accuracy in the lumbar spine, MRI will give more information and a more complete anatomic depiction than will CT. There are a host of things that can be seen on an MRI study that cannot be seen with CT, yet it remains to be seen if the additional information afforded by an MRI examination will prove to be clinically useful. For example, MRI can determine if a disc is degenerated by showing loss of signal on T2-weighted images (Fig. 11-1). CT cannot give this information, but it hardly matters because no treatment is currently given solely for a degenerated disc. In fact, degenerative discs have been reported in asymptomatic children who deny a history of back pain.[5]

IMAGING PROTOCOLS

To achieve a high degree of accuracy it is imperative that the proper imaging protocol be observed. Thin section axial images (4 or 5 mm) should be obtained from the mid-body of L3 to the mid-body of S1. Angling of the plane of imaging to be parallel to the discs is not necessary (Fig. 11-2), and contiguous images without skip areas are considered mandatory (Fig. 11-3). Even though sagittal images will be obtained, a host of entities are more easily identified on the axial images than on the sagittal images. These include migrated free disc fragments,

spondylolysis (pars breaks), conjoined nerve roots, the facets, the neuroforamen, the lateral recesses, and intraspinal synovial cysts. We looked at 103 consecutive spine MRI studies[6] in which we obtained our standard axial and sagittal T1- and T2-weighted sequences; the axial cuts were contiguous, stacked images without gaps or angling. In addition, we obtained axial images that were angled parallel to the discs and covered only the disc spaces, thereby leaving a gap between one level and the next (see Fig. 11-2). The angled axial images were combined with the sagittal images and evaluated for free disc fragments and pars breaks, and then they were compared with the original interpretations, which had the stacked axials and the sagittals. Our standard imaging protocol found 15 cases of spondylolysis and 8 free disc fragments. The angled axial protocol only showed eight cases of spondylolysis and three free fragments, even though the sagittal images were available. We missed three fourths of the free fragments! These patients would likely have all had unsuccessful surgical results with the angled axial protocol. There's no reason I've ever heard of for angling the axial cuts and leaving gaps, yet about a third of all the consult spine cases I look at use this protocol. I think it's the primary cause of missed diagnoses in spine imaging.

Both T1-weighted (or proton density) and T2-weighted (or T2*-weighted) images should be obtained in both the sagittal and the axial planes. Attempts to shorten the study by foregoing one of the T2 sequences was once a popular practice, but it is not recommended. The T2 axial images will increase the diagnostic accuracy and the confidence of many diagnoses.

DISC DISEASE

Terminology plays a large role in how radiologists describe disc bulges or protrusions. Since the

FIGURE 11-1 **Desiccated disc.** A sagittal T2-weighted image shows the L2-3 and L3-4 discs to be abnormally low in signal indicating disc desiccation and degeneration. Compare with the normal L1-2 disc (*arrow*), which has high signal.

FIGURE 11-3 **Proper MRI technique.** This MRI scout with cursors placed contiguously from the body of L3 to S1 allows complete coverage of the lower lumbar spine in the axial plane.

FIGURE 11-2 **Inadequate technique—skip areas.** An MRI scout film with cursors placed through the disc spaces. This allows large gaps or skip areas that can result in multiple missed diagnoses including missed free fragments of discs.

advent of CT in the 1970s, disc bulges have been described by their morphology. A broadbased disc bulge was said to be a bulging annulus fibrosus, whereas a focal disc bulge was called a herniated nucleus pulposus (HNP) (Fig. 11-4). This is no longer the accepted terminology. Although no universally accepted classification of disc disease is present, most agree on something like the following: a broadbased disc bulge is called a bulge; a focal bulge is called a protrusion; a piece of disc that has migrated from the parent disc is a free fragment or sequestration. The term HNP is no longer considered acceptable. More significantly, most surgeons do not care what name is applied to a disc bulge—they do not treat a bulging annulus any differently than a protrusion. They treat the patient's symptoms and have to decide if the disc bulge is responsible for those symptoms. It has been shown in multiple studies that from 10 to 25% of asymptomatic young people have disc bulges or protrusions[7]; hence, just seeing a disc bulge on CT or MRI does not mean it is clinically significant.

MRI has a high degree of accuracy in delineating disc protrusions and showing if neural tissue is impressed (Fig. 11-5). MRI can also show if annu-

BROADBASED   FOCAL

FIGURE 11-4 **Schematic of types of disc bulges.** The broadbased disc bulge (*left*) is typical for a bulging annulus fibrosus. A focal disc bulge (*right*) is more consistent with a protrusion.

A

B

FIGURE 11-5 **Disc protrusions.** An axial T1-weighted image (*A*) shows a focal disc protrusion (*arrows*). An axial gradient echo image (*B*) shows a broadbased disc bulge (*arrows*). Because these are both showing impression of the thecal sac, they could each cause symptoms.

lar fibers of the disc are disrupted (Fig. 11-6)—a so-called extrusion or HIZ (high-intensity zone). Although CT cannot diagnose extrusions, clinicians do not currently treat extrusions any differently than protrusions (annular fibers intact). It is true that an extrusion must be present before a sequestration (free fragment) can occur; however, an extrusion without a free fragment has no more significance than a mere disc bulge. The key question is whether the bulging disc material is impressing neural tissue and causing the patient's symptoms.

Free Fragments

A type of disc extrusion that is critical to diagnose is the free fragment or sequestration. Missed free fragments are one of the most common causes of failed back surgery.[8] The preoperative diagnosis of a free fragment contraindicates chymopapain, percutaneous discectomy, and, for many surgeons, microdiscectomy. At the very least it means the surgeon needs to explore more cephalad or caudally during the surgery to remove the free fragment. As free fragments can be difficult to diagnose clinically, imaging is critical in the evaluation of the spine for any patient contemplating surgery. At times it can be difficult to be absolutely certain as to whether a disc that lies above or below the disc space is still attached to the parent disc or is really "free." So long as disc material is above or below the level of the disc space it really does not matter if it is attached or not—chymopapain and percutaneous discectomy would still be contraindicated and many surgeons would not perform a microdiscectomy (at the very least they would increase their exposure to find and remove the disc fragment). The key element is recognizing that disc material is present away from the level of the disc space.

Free fragments are diagnosed on MRI by noting disc material cephalad or caudal to the disc space (Fig. 11-7). Free fragments may migrate either cranially or caudally with no apparent preference.

Axial images often show the free fragment more conspicuously than the sagittal images (Fig. 11-8); therefore, contiguous axial images without large skip areas or gaps are imperative to avoid missing free fragments.

A conjoined root, which is a normal variant of two roots exiting the thecal sac together or in an anomalous manner (seen in 1 to 3% of the

FIGURE 11-6 **Annular tear.** This sagittal fast spin-echo T2 image shows a focus of increased signal (*arrow*) in the annulus that is called an HIZ (high-intensity zone), which indicates an annular tear.

population)[9] (Fig. 11-9), or a Tarlov cyst, a normal variant in which a nerve root sleeve is dilated, can have a similar appearance to a free fragment but can almost always be differentiated from disc material by their signal staying isointense to the thecal sac on both T1 and T2 sequences. It is critical to identify a conjoined root or a Tarlov cyst and not confuse them for a free fragment. A surgeon will often change his or her procedure and certainly the amount of surgical exploration if he or she thinks there is a free fragment present. Many surgeons have inadvertently damaged conjoined or anomalous nerve roots thinking they were free fragments. Obviously, a free fragment should be removed and a conjoined nerve root should be left alone—the imaging study is where that difference should be ascertained, not during surgery.

Lateral Discs

Discs will occasionally protrude in a lateral direction causing the nerve root that has already exited the central canal to be stretched (Fig. 11-10). Although not common (less than 5% of cases), these are frequently overlooked and are known to be a source of failed back surgery.[10] Because they affect the previously exited root, they can clinically mimic symptoms of a disc protrusion from one level more cephalad (Fig. 11-11). For example, in a patient with multilevel disc disease and symptoms referable to the L3-4 disc, the disc protrusion is usually a posterior L3-4 bulge that impresses the

A   **B**

FIGURE 11-7 **Free fragment.** *A,* A sagittal T1-weighted MR image shows a large amount of disc material bulging posteriorly at the disc space (*arrows*). *B,* The adjacent slice shows disc material that has migrated cephalad (*arrows*) and now lies posterior to the L5 vertebral body. This is a large free fragment.

FIGURE 11-8   **Free fragment more evident on axial images.** The axial image *(A)* reveals an obvious large free disc fragment *(arrow)*, which is causing an obvious distortion of the thecal sac. It is not as conspicuous on the T1-*(B)* or T2-weighted *(C)* sagittal images. The free fragment can be seen posterior to the L3 vertebral body *(arrow)* and is displacing the posterior longitudinal ligament.

FIGURE 11-9   **Conjoined root.** An axial proton density image shows a mass in the right lateral recess that had signal characteristics identical to the thecal sac on all sequences. This is a conjoined nerve root. A free fragment would not have signal identical to the thecal sac on all sequences.

L4 nerve root. However, a lateral disc at L4-5 could impress the L4 nerve root and cause the same symptoms. If unnoticed, surgery could be performed at the L3-4 disc—the wrong level. Unfortunately, I have seen this on several occa-

sions. Also, it is important to notify the surgeon that the disc is lateral to the neuroforamen, because a standard surgical approach through the lamina might not allow removal of a lateral disc.

Lateral discs are best identified on axial images. Sagittal images will often show a lateral disc occluding a neuroforamen, but many times a lateral disc will not extend into the foramen and the sagittal images will appear normal.

STENOSIS

By definition, spinal stenosis is encroachment of the bony or soft tissue structures in the spine on one or more of the neural elements with resulting symptoms. These symptoms are often indistinguishable from those of disc disease, and, in fact, disc disease often coexists with spinal stenosis. Patients with spinal stenosis classically present with back pain and bilateral sciatica, intermittent claudication, pain with hyperextension and relief with flexion, and pain with standing that is relieved by lying down.

Spinal stenosis is classically divided into congenital and acquired types; however, even the most severe forms of congenital stenosis do not cause symptoms unless a component of acquired stenosis (usually degenerative disease of the facets and

A   **B**

FIGURE 11-10   **Lateral disc.** *A,* A sagittal T1-weighted magnetic resonance image through the left neuroforamen shows a low-signal structure in the L4 neuroforamen *(arrow),* which is a lateral disc protrusion. *B,* Axial T1 (upper) and T2* (lower) show the lateral disc *(arrows)* in the left neuroforamen.

FIGURE 11-11 **Schematic of lateral disc.** This schematic illustrates how a posterior L4-5 disc protrusion affects the L5 nerve root, yet a lateral L4-5 disc affects the L4 root.

the discs) is present. A more useful classification of stenosis is on an anatomic basis: central canal, neuroforaminal, and lateral recess. It is important to realize that stenosis and disc disease are often present concomitantly, and it can be difficult to clinically differentiate the two. As with disc disease, it is imperative that any imaging findings be matched with the clinical picture. It is not unusual to have a patient with severe stenosis on an imaging study and no clinical symptoms.

Central Canal Stenosis

Although at one time measurements were considered useful in the determination of central canal stenosis, they are no longer believed to be a valid indicator of disease. Instead, simply noting whether the thecal sac is compressed or round will reliably serve for determining central canal stenosis (Fig. 11-12). A subjective assessment as to whether the compression (usually in an anteroposterior direction) is mild, moderate, or severe is all that is necessary for evaluating the central canal. It is quite common to note mild or moderate central canal stenosis with flattening of the thecal sac in a patient who is asymptomatic.

The most common cause of central canal stenosis is degenerative disease of the facets with bony hypertrophy, which encroaches on the central canal (Fig. 11-13). This is also the most common cause of lateral recess stenosis. When the facets undergo degenerative joint disease (DJD) they often have some slippage, which results in buckling of the ligamentum flavum. Although a misnomer, this has been termed ligamentum flavum hypertrophy and is a common cause of central canal stenosis (Fig. 11-14). Frequently, mild disc bulging is associated with minimal facet hypertrophy and ligamentum flavum hypertrophy. This combination can result in severe focal central canal stenosis.

FIGURE 11-12 **Central canal stenosis.** An axial T1-weighted image shows compression of the thecal sac in an anteroposterior direction, which is diagnostic of central canal stenosis.

FIGURE 11-13 **Facet hypertrophy causing stenosis.** This MR image shows marked facet degenerative disease with hypertrophy of the facets causing lateral recess and central canal stenosis.

Less common causes of central canal stenosis include bony overgrowth from Paget's disease, achondroplasia, posttraumatic changes, and severe spondylolisthesis.

Neuroforaminal Stenosis

DJD of the facets with bony hypertrophy is the most common cause of neuroforaminal stenosis;

FIGURE 11-14 **Ligamentum flavum hypertrophy.** Inward bulging of the ligamentum flavum (*arrows*) is shown on this MR image. Central canal stenosis from ligamentum flavum hypertrophy is common.

FIGURE 11-15 **Normal neuroforamen.** A sagittal T1-weighted image through the neuroforamen shows the nerve roots surrounded by fat with no evidence of foraminal stenosis. This does not exclude, however, a focus of foraminal stenosis that is medial or lateral to this sagittal image.

however, encroachment on the nerve root in the neuroforamen can be seen with free disc fragments, postoperative scar, and from a lateral disc protrusion.

The neuroforamen is best evaluated on axial images just cephalad to the disc space. The disc space lies at the inferior portion of the neuroforamen, and the exiting nerve root lies in the superior or cephalad portion of the neuroforamen. Although the neuroforamen can be clearly seen on sagittal MR images (Fig. 11-15), care must be taken to evaluate the entire neuroforamen and not just the 4 or 5 mm of one sagittal image. A normal-appearing neuroforamen on a sagittal image does not exclude neuroforaminal stenosis (the axial images must be evaluated), whereas a stenotic foramen seen on a sagittal image (Fig. 11-16) can be counted on as being reliable for pathology.

Lateral Recess Stenosis

The lateral recesses are the bony canals in which the nerve roots lie after they leave the thecal sac and before they enter the neuroforamen. The lateral recesses are bounded by the neuroforamen caudally and cranially. They are triangular in shape when viewed on axial images, and the nerve root can be identified as a low-signal rounded structure on all imaging sequences. Hypertrophy of the superior articular facet from DJD is the most common cause of encroachment on the lateral recesses

FIGURE 11-16 **Neuroforaminal stenosis.** Marked narrowing of the neuroforamen (*arrow*) is seen on this sagittal T1-weighted image.

(Fig. 11-17), although, as with the neuroforamen, disc fragments and postoperative scarring can cause nerve root impingement.

POSTOPERATIVE CHANGES

Failed back surgery, unfortunately, is common. It can occur from many causes, including inade-

FIGURE 11-17 **Lateral recess stenosis.** Hypertrophy of the right-sided facet with encroachment into the lateral recess (*arrow*) is seen on this drawing.

quate surgery (including missed free disc fragments), postoperative scarring, failure of bone grafting for fusion, and recurrent disc protrusion. CT is useful in evaluating bone grafts but is not reliable for differentiating postoperative scarring

from disc material. MRI has been shown to be particularly useful in distinguishing scar from disc material.

The use of intravenous gadolinium will allow virtual certainty in distinguishing scar from disc. Scar tissue will be enhanced after administration of gadolinium, whereas disc material will have only some minimal peripheral enhancement, presumably caused by inflammation (Fig. 11-18).

BONY ABNORMALITIES

Spondylolysis and Spondylolisthesis

Defects in the bony pars interarticularis (spondylolysis) are commonly found in asymptomatic individuals, yet they can be a source of low back pain and instability. Before disc surgery or other back surgery, it is imperative that any spondylolysis be identified. Because spondylolysis can mimic back pain from other pathology, it is important to assess it before surgery. If necessary, it can then be surgically addressed at the same time as the other surgery. Failure to note and evaluate spondylolysis is a known source of failed back surgery.

A   **B**

FIGURE 11-18 **Postoperative scar enhancement with gadolinium.** *A,* A T1-weighted axial image shows scar tissue surrounding the thecal sac and makes evaluation for recurrent disc protrusion difficult. *B,* A T1-weighted axial image through the same level after administration of gadolinium intravenously shows enhancement of the scar tissue surrounding the thecal sac. No significant disc protrusion can be identified.

FIGURE 11-19 **Spondylolysis**. An axial T2-weighted image through the mid-vertebral body reveals a break in the bony laminae bilaterally (*arrows*), which indicates spondylolysis. An axial cut through the pedicles should have an intact bony ring around the central canal.

FIGURE 11-20   **Type 2 marrow changes**. A sagittal T1-weighted image in a patient with degenerative disc disease shows bands of fatty marrow parallel to the L4-5 end-plates (*arrows*), which are type 2 marrow changes often seen with degenerative disc disease.

CT is superior to MRI at identifying spondylolysis.[11] Although MRI will show spondylolysis defects, they can be difficult to see at times. As previously mentioned, this is the only area in which CT is reported to be clearly superior to MRI in evaluating the lumbar spine. Spondylolysis is identified on the axial images through the mid-vertebral body as a break in the normally intact bony ring of the lamina (Fig. 11-19). A protocol using axial images only through the discs will routinely miss spondylolysis defects. Care must be used in calling spondylolysis on the sagittal views as the normal pars often has a low signal area that resembles spondylolysis. If the pars appears normal on the sagittal view, it can be considered a reliable finding; however, if the pars appears abnormal on the sagittal view, the axial view must be used to determine if a break is really present.

Spondylolisthesis (forward slippage of one vertebral body on a lower one) occurs from either slippage of two vertebral bodies after bilateral spondylolysis or from DJD of the facets with slippage of the facets. Bilateral spondylolysis can result in a large amount of slippage, whereas facet DJD will usually result in only minimal slippage. If spondylolisthesis is severe, it can result in central canal stenosis, neuroforaminal stenosis, or both.

End-plate Changes

Parallel bands of high or low signal adjacent to the vertebral body end-plates are often seen in association with degenerative disc disease. The most common appearance is of high-signal bands on T1-weighted images that remain high on T2-weighted images (Fig. 11-20). This represents fatty marrow conversion. It was seen in 16% of cases in the first report by Modic and colleagues[1] and was termed type 2 changes (generally referred to as "Modic type 2"). Modic type 1 changes are seen as low-signal bands parallel to the end-plates on T1-weighted images that get brighter on T2-weighted images (Fig. 11-21). This represents an inflammatory or granulomatous response to degenerative disc disease. The type 1 changes were reported in 4% of cases and must be distinguished from disc space infection (Fig. 11-22). In disc space infection the disc should get bright on the T2-weighted images, whereas it is unusual for a degenerative disc to have high signal on T2-weighted images. Modic type 3 changes are parallel

A   B

FIGURE 11-21   **Type 1 marrow changes.** *A,* A sagittal T1-weighted image in a patient with degenerative disc disease at L3-4 shows faint bands of low signal parallel to the L3-4 end-plates *(arrows)*. *B,* A sagittal fast spin-echo T2-weighted image with fat suppression shows bands of high signal adjacent to the L3-4 end-plates. This represents granulation tissue seen with degenerative disc disease and has been called type 1 marrow change. It can be differentiated from a disc infection by the low signal of the disc on the T2-weighted image.

A   **B**

FIGURE 11-22   **Disc infection.** *A,* A sagittal T1-weighted image shows bands of low signal in the vertebral bodies adjacent to the L4-5 end-plates. On a T2-weighted (gradient-echo) image (*B*) the vertebral body/end-plate signal increase is faintly seen as it is a gradient-echo sequence. However, note the high signal in the disc, which makes this consistent with a disc infection rather than a type 2 signal of a degenerative disc.

bands of low signal adjacent to the end-plates on both T1- and T2-weighted images. Type 3 changes represent bony sclerosis seen on plain films.

REFERENCES

1. Modic M, Masaryk T, Ross J, Carter J: Imaging of degenerative disk disease. Radiology 1988;168:177-186.
2. Hesselink J: Spine imaging: History, achievements, remaining frontiers. AJR 1988;150:1223-1230.
3. Jackson R, Becker G, Jacobs R, et al: The neuroradiographic diagnosis of lumbar herniated nucleus pulposus (I): A comparison of computed tomography, myelography, CT-myelography, discography, and CT-discography. Spine 1989;14:1356-1361.
4. Jackson R, Cain J, Jacobs R, et al: The neuroradiographic diagnosis of lumbar herniated nucleus pulposus (II): A comparison of computed tomography, myelography, CT-myelography, and magnetic resonance imaging. Spine 1989;14:1362-1367.
5. Tertti M, Salminen J, Paajanen H, et al: Low-back pain and disk degeneration in children: A case-control MR imaging study. Radiology 1991;180:503-507.
6. Fiorella D, Jones T, Helms CA, et al: Angled axial MR images in the lumbar spine: A potential source of diagnostic error. Radiology 1999;213(P):157.
7. Jensen MC, Brant-Zawadzki MN, Obuchowski N, et al: Abnormal magnetic-resonance scans of the lumbar spine in asymptomatic subjects. NEJM 1994; 331:69-73.
8. Onik G, Mooney V, Maroon J, et al: Automated percutaneous discectomy: A prospective multi-institutional study. Neurosurgery 1989;26:228-233.
9. Helms CA, Dorwart RH, Gray M: The CT appearance of conjoined nerve roots and differentiation from a herniated nucleus pulposus. Radiology 1982;144:803-807.
10. Winter DDB, Munk PL, Helms CA, et al: CT and MR of lateral disc herniation: Typical appearance and pitfalls of interpretation. J Can Assoc Radiol 1989;40:256-259.
11. Grenier N, Kressel HY, Schiebler ML, Grossman RI: Isthmic spondylolysis of the lumbar spine: MR imaging at 1.5 T. Radiology 1989;170:489-494.

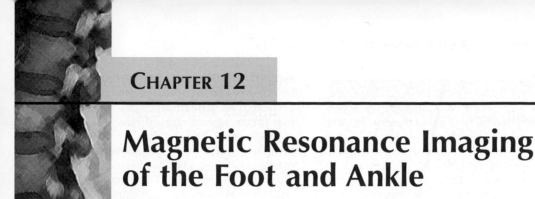

CHAPTER 12

Magnetic Resonance Imaging of the Foot and Ankle

I have always found topics on the foot and ankle to be exceedingly boring. This is mainly because I was never called on to use any of the information I learned; hence, I quickly forgot all that I was told. I learned early in my residency that during lectures on the foot and ankle I could find better use of my time—like running or playing golf. That has changed now that magnetic resonance imaging (MRI) is being used in the foot and ankle. MRI is playing an increasingly important role in examining the foot and ankle. Orthopedic surgeons and podiatrists are learning that critical diagnostic information can be obtained in no other way and are relying on MRI for many therapeutic decisions.

When most of us first encounter an ankle MR image, we get out a cross-sectional atlas and start trying to determine where all the tendons, muscles, vascular structures, and so on lie. I can assure you this will be unnecessary after reading this chapter. Although the anatomy of the foot and ankle can be complex, the significant anatomy, that is, the anatomy that must be learned because it is affected by disease, is fairly straightforward and easily learned.[1] There is no need to memorize tendons, ligaments, and muscles that are only rarely seen to be abnormal; therefore, this chapter will dwell only on the pathologically significant areas.

I must admit, imaging the foot and ankle is getting more complex. It seems there is a new article every month on the utility of MRI in this area. Foot and ankle imaging is one of the fastest growing studies in musculoskeletal imaging, and this chapter has the most significant number of changes compared with the previous edition.

TENDONS

One of the more common reasons to perform an MRI examination on the foot and ankle is to examine the tendons. Although multiple tendons course through the ankle, only a few are routinely affected pathologically. These are primarily the flexor tendons, located posteriorly in the ankle. The extensor tendons, located anteriorly, are rarely abnormal.

Tendons can be directly traumatized or can be injured from overuse. Either etiologic factor can result in the following conditions: *tenosynovitis,* which is seen on MRI as fluid in the tendon sheath with the underlying tendon appearing normal; *tendonitis* or a partial tear, which is seen as focal or fusiform swelling of the tendon with signal within the tendon that gets bright on T2 or T2* images; thinning or attenuation of the tendon is a more severe form of tendonitis, often presaging a tendon rupture; and *tendon rupture,* which is best identified on axial images by noting absence of a tendon on one or more images.

Making the distinction between tenosynovitis and tendonitis is not crucial because the treatment is similar for both entities. However, it is important to distinguish between tendonitis and a complete disruption because surgical repair is often warranted for the latter and not for the former. It is often difficult to make the distinction clinically.

Complete tendon disruption can be difficult to see on sagittal or coronal images because of the tendency for tendons to course obliquely to the plane of imaging. An exception to this is the Achilles tendon, which is usually best seen on a sagittal image. The imaging protocol for the foot and ankle must include axial images with T1 (or proton density) and T2 (or T2*) sequences. It is not recommended that both ankles be studied together. An extremity coil around one ankle with a small field of view will give the highest image quality. A sagittal image with both T1 and T2 weighting is also performed but can be replaced with images in the coronal plane in some cases depending on the preference of the radiologist.

Achilles Tendon. The Achilles tendon does not have a sheath associated with it; therefore, tenosynovitis does not occur. Tendonitis (or, if you prefer, tendinosis) is commonly seen in the Achilles; however, it is such an easy clinical diagnosis that MRI is usually not necessary. Complete disruption is commonly seen in athletes and in men around the age of 40. It is also commonly associated with other systemic disorders that cause tendon weakening, such as rheumatoid arthritis, collagen vascular diseases, crystal deposition diseases, and hyperparathyroidism.

Achilles tendon disruption can be treated surgically or by placing the patient in a cast with equinus positioning (marked plantar flexion) for several months. It is controversial as to which treatment is superior, with both methods of treatment seemingly working well. I have known two surgeons who were dogmatic in their approach to always recommending surgery for torn Achilles tendons until they ruptured their own and opted for nonsurgical treatment.

MRI is being used by some surgeons to help decide if surgery should be performed. If a large gap is present (Fig. 12-1), some surgeons feel surgery should be performed to reappose the torn ends of the tendon; whereas if the ends of the tendon are not retracted, nonsurgical treatment is preferred. No articles have been published to show that this is, in fact, scientifically valid.

Posterior Tibial Tendon. The flexor tendons are easily remembered and identified by using the mnemonic "Tom, Dick, and Harry," with Tom representing the posterior Tibial tendon (PTT), Dick the flexor Digitorum longus, and Harry the flexor Hallucis longus (FHL) (Fig. 12-2). The PTT is the most medial and the largest, with the exception of the Achilles, of the flexor tendons. The PTT inserts onto the navicular, second and third cuneiforms, and the bases of the second to fourth metatarsals. As it sweeps under the foot, it provides some support for the longitudinal arch; hence, problems in the arch or plantar fascia can sometimes lead to stress on the PTT with resulting tendonitis or even rupture. Posterior tibial tendonitis and rupture are commonly encountered in rheumatoid arthritis.

Rupture of the PTT results clinically in a flat foot because of the loss of arch support given by this tendon. The spring ligament runs just deep to the PTT and then goes underneath the neck of the talus, which it supports in a slinglike fashion. When the PTT tears, the stress is then placed on the spring ligament to support the talus and the arch. The spring ligament has a high incidence of disruption when the PTT tears. Once the PTT and the spring ligament tear, the next structure to fail is the subtalar joint ligaments—the sinus tarsi. We looked at 25 patients with PTT tears and found that 92% of the cases had abnormal spring ligaments (thickened or torn) and 72% had an abnormal sinus tarsi.[2] It's clear these structures are linked, and injury or stress to one can affect the others.

Differentiation of tendonitis (many consider the use of the term tendonitis to be inappropriate and have replaced it with tendinosis; whatever) from tendon rupture can be difficult clinically, and MRI has become valuable for making this distinction.[3] Most surgeons will operate on a disrupted PTT, whereas nonoperative therapy is usually preferred for tendonitis.

Posterior tibial tendonitis is seen on axial T1-weighted images as swelling and/or signal within the normally low-signal tendon on one or more images (Fig. 12-3). T2 or T2* images show the signal in the tendon getting brighter. Tendon disruption is diagnosed by noting the absence of low-signal tendon on one or more axial images (Fig. 12-4). This typically occurs just at or above the level of the tibiotalar joint.

The spring ligament is identified on axial and coronal images just deep to the PTT. When it is stressed, it typically gets scarred and thickened (Fig. 12-5). A tear can be diagnosed by noting a gap in the ligament.

FIGURE 12-1 **Torn Achilles tendon.** A sagittal T1-weighted image reveals the Achilles tendon to be torn with a 2-cm gap. Only a thin remnant of the tendon remains intact across the gap (*arrow*). Note the high signal in the swollen ends of the separated tendon, indicative of hemorrhage and edema.

FIGURE 12-3 **Posterior tibial tendon tendonitis.** A proton density axial image through the ankle at the level of the mid-calcaneus shows the posterior tibial tendon (*arrow*) swollen and containing high signal. This is the appearance of marked tendonitis.

FIGURE 12-2 **Normal ankle anatomy.** *A,* This drawing of the tendons around the ankle at the level of the tibiotalar joint shows the relation of the flexor tendons posteriorly and the extensor tendons anteriorly. *B,* An axial T1-weighted image through the ankle just above the tibiotalar joint shows the normal anatomy. A, Achilles tendon; D, flexor digitorum tendon; H, flexor hallucis tendon; P, peroneal tendons; T, posterior tibial tendon; TA, tibialis anterior tendon.

Flexor Hallucis Longus. The FHL tendon is easily identified near the tibiotalar joint because it is usually the only tendon at that distal level that has muscle still attached. In the foot the FHL is easily identified beneath the sustentaculum talus, which it uses as a pulley to plantar flex the foot.

The FHL is known as the Achilles tendon of the foot in ballet dancers because of the extreme flexion position they frequently use. Ballet dancers often will have tenosynovitis of the FHL, seen on MRI as fluid in the sheath surrounding the tendon. Care must be taken to have clinical correlation, because up to 20% of people in general have a communication between the ankle joint and the FHL tendon sheath; therefore, fluid can be seen in the FHL tendon sheath from a connection to an ankle joint, which has an effusion. Rupture of the FHL is rare.

Peroneal Tendons. The peroneus longus and brevis tendons can be seen posterior to the distal fibula, to which they are bound by a thin fibrous structure, the superior retinaculum. The fibula serves as a pulley for the tendons to work as the principal everter of the foot. The tendons course close together adjacent to the lateral aspect of the calcaneus until a few centimeters below the lateral malleolus where they separate, with the peroneus brevis inserting onto the base of the fifth metatarsal and the peroneus longus crossing under the foot to the base of the first metatarsal. Avulsion of the base of the fifth metatarsal from a pull by the peroneus brevis is known as a "dancer's fracture" or a Jones fracture.

A

B

FIGURE 12-4 **Torn posterior tibial tendon.** Axial T1- (*A*) and T2-weighted (*B*) images through the ankle in this patient with chronic pain reveal a distended posterior tibial tendon sheath (*arrows*) with no low-signal tendon identified within. This is a tear of the posterior tibial tendon.

Disruption of the superior retinaculum, often seen in skiing accidents, can result in displacement of the peroneal tendons (Fig. 12-6), which must be surgically corrected. It often occurs with a small bony avulsion, called a flake fracture, off of the fibula caused by the avulsed superior retinaculum.

FIGURE 12-5 **Abnormal spring ligament.** An axial T2-weighted image through the ankle shows a markedly thickened spring ligament (*arrows*) just deep to the posterior tibial tendon.

Entrapment of the peroneal tendons in a fractured calcaneus or fibula can occur and is easily diagnosed with MR. This can be a difficult diagnosis to make clinically. Complete disruption of the peroneals is uncommon, but it is easily noted with MR.

Longitudinal split tears of the peroneus brevis are commonly seen in patients after an inversion ankle sprain with associated dorsiflexion. The peroneus brevis gets trapped against the fibula by the peroneus longus and a longitudinal split tear of the peroneus brevis results. These patients have chronic lateral ankle pain, often associated with ankle instability caused by the lateral collateral ligament disruption that also occurs with the inversion trauma. A split tear of the peroneus brevis is easily identified on MRI by noting either a chevron or "V" shape to the tendon distal to the fibula (Fig. 12-7), or noting a division of the tendon into two parts. There is an 80% association with lateral ligament tears, therefore close attention should be paid to the ligaments when a split tear of the peroneus brevis is found.

AVASCULAR NECROSIS

Avascular necrosis (AVN) commonly occurs in the foot and ankle. The talar dome is the second most common location of osteochondritis dissecans (the knee is the most common site). MRI is useful in identifying and staging osteochondritis dissecans (which, for whatever reason, is now called an osteochondral lesion [OCL]). Even when not apparent on plain films, MRI can show an OCL as a focal area of low signal in the subarticular portion of the talar dome on T1-weighted images. On T2 or T2* images, if high signal is seen surrounding the OCL fragment, in the bone at the bed of the fragment, or throughout the fragment (Fig. 12-8), it is most likely an unstable fragment. If the fragment has become displaced and lies in the joint as

FIGURE 12-6 **Dislocated peroneus longus tendon.** An axial T1-weighted image in this rock climber who injured his ankle in a fall shows a low-signal rounded structure (*arrow*) lateral to the lateral malleolus. This is a dislocated peroneus longus tendon.

A

B

FIGURE 12-8 **Unstable osteochondritis dissecans of the talus.** *A,* A proton density coronal image through the talus shows a focus of low signal in the medial subarticular part of the talus (*arrow*). This is a characteristic appearance for osteochondritis dissecans. *B,* A T2-weighted image shows high signal throughout the focus of osteochondritis dissecans, which indicates an unstable fragment.

FIGURE 12-7 **Longitudinal split tear of the peroneus brevis.** This axial T1-weighted image shows the peroneus brevis (*arrow*) with a "V" or chevron shape, which is characteristic for a longitudinal split tear of the brevis.

a loose body, MRI can sometimes be useful in localizing it; however, loose bodies in any joint can be exceedingly difficult to find.

Diffuse low signal throughout a tarsal bone on T1- and T2-weighted images is typical for AVN. If the T2-weighted images have increased signal throughout, it may or may not be reversible. This occasionally occurs in the tarsal navicular (Fig. 12-9). MRI can be useful in making this diagnosis when plain films are normal or equivocal. AVN in the tarsal navicular can result from continued weight bearing on a fracture that was not diagnosed. This is often seen in athletes, especially basketball players, and can be a career-ending injury in a professional athlete.

TUMORS

There are a few tumors that have a predilection for the foot and ankle.[4] Up to 16% of synovial sarcomas occur in the foot. Desmoid tumors are commonly seen in the foot. Giant cell tumors of tendon sheath are often found in the tendon sheaths of the foot and ankle (Fig. 12-10). They are characterized by marked low signal in the synovial lining and in the tendons on T1 and T2 images, similar to the appearance of PVNS in a joint.

The differential diagnosis for calcaneal tumors is similar to that of the epiphyses: giant cell tumor, chondroblastoma, infection—and, in addition, a unicameral bone cyst (Fig. 12-11).

Soft tissue tumors in the medial aspect of the foot and ankle can press on the posterior tibial nerve resulting in tarsal tunnel syndrome.[5] Clinically, patients with tarsal tunnel syndrome have pain and paresthesia in the plantar aspect of the foot. In the aforementioned mnemonic, "Tom,

A

B

FIGURE 12-10   **Giant cell tumor of tendon sheath.** Axial proton density (*A*) and T2-weighted (*B*) images reveal a mass surrounding the flexor hallucis longus tendon (*arrow*), which is confined by the tendon sheath. Although high-signal fluid is present, large amounts of low-signal material is lining the distended tendon sheath. This low signal is hemosiderin, which is typically found in a giant cell tendon of tendon sheath. Pigmented villonodular synovitis in a joint has an identical appearance.

FIGURE 12-9   **Avascular necrosis of the tarsal navicular.** A T1-weighted sagittal image of the ankle in this patient with pain on the dorsum of the foot shows diffuse low signal throughout the tarsal navicular. This is a characteristic appearance for avascular necrosis and will often precede any plain film findings.

FIGURE 12-11 Calcaneal unicameral bone cyst. A T1-weighted axial image through the calcaneus reveals a typical unicameral bone cyst. Note that some fatty material is present in the periphery and fluid is present in the central portion. Biopsy of the peripheral portion could lead to an erroneous diagnosis of an intraosseous lipoma. Unicameral bone cysts will occasionally have fatty elements within, as well as serous fluid.

FIGURE 12-12 Ganglion causing tarsal tunnel syndrome. A T2-weighted axial image of the ankle in a patient describing pain and paresthesia on the plantar aspect of the foot shows a high-signal mass (*arrow*) lying adjacent to the flexor hallucis longus tendon. This is the position of the posterior tibial nerve that can be impinged by a mass, such as in this case, resulting in tarsal tunnel syndrome. This was a ganglion.

Dick, and Harry," the "and" is for artery, nerve, and vein. It is the position of the posterior tibial nerve. The nerve is easily compressed in the tarsal tunnel, which is bounded medially by the flexor retinaculum—a strong fibrous band that extends across the medial ankle joint for about 5 to 7 cm in a superior to inferior direction. Ganglions and neural tumors, both of which can look similar on T1- and T2-weighted images, often lie in the tarsal tunnel (Fig. 12-12) and compress the posterior tibial nerve, resulting in pain and paresthesia on the plantar aspect of the foot extending into the toes. Tarsal tunnel syndrome often occurs secondary to trauma, fibrosis, or idiopathically, all of which may not respond to surgical intervention; hence, MRI is valuable in delineating a treatable lesion in many cases. An MRI examination for tarsal tunnel syndrome is becoming increasingly requested as surgeons learn how valuable it can be in identifying the source of the symptoms.

Anomalous muscles in the foot or ankle are reported to be present in up to 6% of the population.

These can be mistaken for a tumor and a biopsy may be performed unnecessarily. MRI will show these "tumors" to have imaging characteristics identical to normal muscle (Fig. 12-13) and to be sharply circumscribed. Accessory soleus and peroneus quartus muscles are the most common accessory muscles encountered around the foot and ankle.

LIGAMENTS

MRI is not the best way to diagnose acute ankle ligament abnormalities. The clinical evaluation is usually straightforward, and no diagnostic imaging of any type is necessary. Nevertheless, in clinically equivocal cases, when the examination is ordered for other reasons, or in cases of chronic lateral ankle pain, the ligaments can be clearly evaluated with high-quality MRI.[6]

The deltoid ligament lies medially as a broad band beneath the medial flexor tendons. It can be seen extending from the medial malleolus to the talus and calcaneus. It has multiple parts that are

FIGURE 12-13 **Anomalous muscle.** An axial T1-weighted image of both ankles in this patient describing a mass in the right ankle shows an anomalous muscle (*arrow*) lateral to the flexor hallucis longus muscle, which is responsible for the mass that the patient feels.

not easily separated with MRI. It is considered injured when it has increased T2 signal.

The lateral collateral ligament complex is responsible for more than 90% of all ankle ligament injuries. It is made up of two parts: a superior group, the anterior and posterior tib-fib ligaments that make up part of the syndesmosis (Fig. 12-14); and an inferior group, the anterior and posterior talofibular ligaments and the calcaneofibular ligament (Fig. 12-15). The anterior and posterior tib-fib ligaments can be seen on axial images at the level of the dome of the talus. The anterior and posterior talofibular ligaments are seen on the axial images just below the tibiotalar

joint and emanate from a concavity in the distal fibula called the malleolar fossa (see Fig. 12-15B). The most commonly torn ankle ligament is the anterior talofibular ligament. It is easily identified when a joint effusion is present because it makes up the anterior capsule of the joint (Fig. 12-16). The anterior talofibular ligament is usually torn without other ligaments being involved; however, if the injury is severe enough, the next ligament to tear is the calcaneofibular ligament. Even with severe trauma, the posterior talofibular ligament rarely tears. The calcaneofibular and posterior talofibular ligaments will not be torn without a tear of the anterior talofibular ligament.

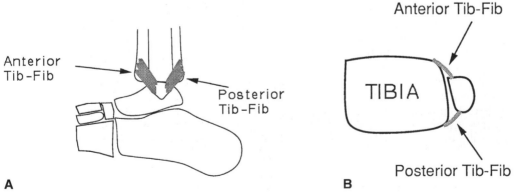

FIGURE 12-14 **Schematic of lateral collateral ligaments.** This drawing of the ankle in a lateral view (*A*) shows how the anterior and posterior tib-fib ligaments extend off of the fibula and course superiorly to the tibia. A drawing in the axial plane (*B*) shows that the fibula has a flat or convex surface at the origin of these ligaments.

A

B

FIGURE 12-15 **Schematic of lateral collateral ligaments.** This drawing of the ankle in a lateral view (*A*) shows how the anterior and posterior talofibular ligaments and the calcaneofibular ligament extend off of the fibula and course inferiorly. These ligaments arise off of the fibula more distally than the anterior and posterior tib-fib ligaments. A drawing in the axial plane (*B*) shows that the anterior and posterior talofibular ligaments arise from the level of the distal fibula, which has a concave medial surface, the malleolar fossa.

A

B

FIGURE 12-16 **Anterior talofibular ligament.** *A*, An axial T2-weighted image through the distal fibula at the level of the malleolar fossa (the concave medial surface of the fibula) shows an intact anterior talofibular ligament (*arrow*), which makes up part of the joint capsule at this level. Note the high-signal joint fluid adjacent to the ligament. *B*, This axial T2-weighted image at the level of the malleolar fossa reveals a thickened anterior talofibular ligament (*arrow*). The marked thickening of the ligament indicates a chronic process.

Sinus Tarsi Syndrome

An entity that has a high association with torn lateral collateral ligaments in the ankle is sinus tarsi syndrome. Clinically, these patients have lateral ankle pain and a feeling of hindfoot instability. Up to 80% of these patients have torn lateral collateral ligaments and up to one third of patients who tear their lateral collateral ligaments have been reported to have sinus tarsi syndrome.[7] In the past diagnosis has relied on clinical suspicion and injection of Xylocaine into the sinus tarsus, which causes resolution of the pain. Treatment is varied but can include a joint fusion.

The sinus tarsi is the space that lies between the talus and the calcaneus and opens up in a conelike configuration to the lateral aspect of the ankle beneath the lateral malleolus. It is filled with fat and several ligaments that give some hindfoot stability. The most lateral of these ligaments are slips of ligaments from the lateral extensor retinaculum. Medial to these are the cervical ligament, and the most medial ligament is the interosseous ligament (Fig. 12-17). In sinus tarsi syndrome the fat in the sinus tarsus is obliterated and one or more of the ligaments are disrupted (Fig. 12-18). This syndrome is causing an increasing amount of MRI requests as surgeons and podiatrists recognize that a definitive diagnosis of sinus tarsi syndrome can be made with imaging.

BONY ABNORMALITIES

Tarsal coalition is a common cause of a painful flat foot. It occurs most commonly at the calcaneonavicular joint and the middle facet of the talocalcaneal joint (Fig. 12-19). Up to 50% of patients with tarsal coalition have bilateral coalition. It can be difficult (or impossible) to see the coalition on plain films; however CT and MRI will show bony coalition with a high degree of accuracy. The coalition, however, can also be fibrous or cartilaginous.

A

B

FIGURE 12-18   Sinus tarsi syndrome. A sagittal T1-weighted image (*A*) shows obliteration of the normal fat in the sinus tarsi. No ligaments are visualized. A sagittal T2-weighted image (*B*) reveals no evidence of the normal cervical or interosseous ligaments. The high signal throughout the sinus tarsi represents scar or fibrosis. These findings are classic for sinus tarsi syndrome.

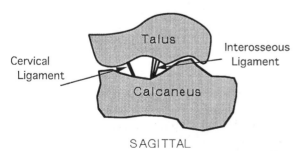

SAGITTAL

FIGURE 12-17   Schematic of the sinus tarsi. A sagittal schematic of the sinus tarsi shows the positions of the cervical and the interosseous ligaments. The cervical ligament lies more anteriorly and laterally in relation to the interosseous ligament.

In these cases, secondary findings, such as joint space irregularity at the affected joint or degenerative joint disease (DJD) at nearby joints that are subjected to accentuated stress, can be seen. For now, MRI does not appear to have superiority to CT for diagnosing tarsal coalition.

Fractures of the foot and ankle are usually well documented with plain films. Stress fractures, however, can be difficult to radiographically or clinically diagnose and can mimic more sinister abnormalities. MRI will show stress fractures as linear low signal on T1-weighted images with high signal on T2 weighting (Fig. 12-20).

MRI has had mixed reviews when used for diagnosing osteomyelitis in the foot. In patients with diabetes who have foot infections, it is important to diagnose osteomyelitis, because the treatment is often much more aggressive, including amputation,

FIGURE 12-19 **Tarsal coalition.** An axial T1-weighted image in a patient with painful flat feet shows bilateral talocalcaneal coalition (*arrows*), which is primarily fibrous. The joint space is irregular and widened bilaterally. In cases of suspected coalition both ankles should be imaged because coalition often occurs bilaterally.

A

B

FIGURE 12-20 **Calcaneal stress fracture.** A 70-year-old woman with a prior history of lung cancer presented with heel pain and a normal plain film (*A*). A bone scan showed diffuse increased radionuclide uptake throughout the posterior calcaneus. A sagittal T1-weighted MR image (*B*) revealed a linear area of low signal (*arrows*), which is characteristic for a stress fracture. Metastatic disease would not have this appearance.

than if the bone is not involved. If the marrow appears normal, MRI is useful in predicting no osteomyelitis; however, if abnormal signal is present in the marrow around a joint, osteomyelitis may or may not be present. Abnormal signal can be caused by edema or hyperemia without infection. The only definitive MR findings for osteomyelitis are cortical disruption, a bony abscess (not a common finding) (Fig. 12-21), or a sinus track (an even less common finding). MRI is therefore very sensitive but not very specific in diagnosing osteomyelitis in the foot and ankle.[8]

CHRONIC LATERAL ANKLE PAIN

Chronic lateral ankle pain is, after the diabetic foot with infection, the bane of most foot and ankle specialists. There are many causes of chronic lateral ankle pain, including DJD, loose bodies, and an OCL of the talus; however, there are four common entities that are easily identified with MRI (Table 12-1). Newer surgical techniques are evolving to treat these entities; however, when several of these occur simultaneously (which is not uncommon), it can be difficult to determine from the clinical examination where the abnormality lies. MRI is useful in helping determine exactly where the pathology is, which then allows the surgeon to direct his therapy more precisely.[9]

Injury to the anterior talofibular ligament from an inversion ankle sprain is the common thread running through all of these diagnoses, being associated in around 80% in each entity. These four entities should be looked for in every ankle MR because they are commonly found even in only minimally symptomatic patients.

Isolated chronic injury to the anterior talofibular ligament may be a cause of chronic lateral ankle

A   **B**

FIGURE 12-21   **Abscess in osteomyelitis.** A coronal T1-weighted image *(A)* of the knee in a patient with a prior amputation shows an area of low signal in the tibia that is worrisome for infection. The corresponding T2-weighted image *(B)* shows an abscess *(arrows)*, which is diagnostic for osteomyelitis.

pain, or it may be only one part of the problem. An 80% association with sinus tarsi syndrome and longitudinal split tears (both of which were discussed earlier in this chapter) has been reported,

TABLE 12-1   **Common Causes of Chronic Lateral Ankle Pain**

Anterior talofibular ligament disruption or scarring
Sinus tarsi syndrome
Longitudinal split tears of the peroneus brevis
Anterolateral impingement

either of which can be a cause of chronic lateral ankle pain by themselves.

Another cause of chronic lateral ankle pain that has a high association with chronic disruption of the anterior talofibular ligament is anterolateral impingement or lateral gutter syndrome. The lateral gutter is simply the lateral joint space between the distal tibia and talus medially and the fibula and lateral collateral ligaments laterally. The synovium gets thickened and scarred from an inversion ankle injury and causes a painful, mechanical block to dorsiflexion. It is easily identified with MRI by noting low-signal scar tissue in the joint just deep to the anterior talofibular ligament where one should see joint fluid (Fig. 12-22).

A   **B**

Figure 12-22   **Anterolateral impingement.** This axial T1-weighted image through the ankle (*A*) reveals absence of the anterior talofibular ligament (*arrow*). The corresponding T2-weighted image (*B*) shows low-signal scar tissue deep to the expected location of the anterior talofibular ligament (*arrow*), which indicates anterolateral impingement syndrome.

REFERENCES

1. Kneeland J, Macrandar S, Middleton W, et al: MR imaging of the normal ankle: Correlation with anatomic sections. AJR Am J Roentgenol 1988;151: 117-126.
2. Balen PF, Helms CA: Association of posterior tibial tendon injury with spring ligament injury, sinus tarsi abnormality, and plantar fasciitis on MR imaging. AJR Am J Roentgenol 2001;176:1137-1143.
3. Rosenberg Z, Cheung Y, Jahss M, et al: Rupture of posterior tibial tendons: CT and MR imaging with surgical correlation. Radiology 1988;169:229-236.
4. Keigley B, Haggar A, Gaba A, et al: Primary tumors of the foot: MR imaging. Radiology 1989;171:755-759.
5. Erickson S, Quinn S, Kneeland J, et al: MR imaging of the tarsal tunnel and related spaces: Normal and abnormal findings with anatomic correlation. AJR Am J Roentgenol 1990;155:323-328.
6. Erickson S, Smith J, Ruiz M, et al: MR imaging of the lateral collateral ligament of the ankle. AJR Am J Roentgenol 1991;156:131-136.
7. Klein M, Spreitzer A: MR imaging of the tarsal sinus and canal: Normal anatomy, pathologic findings, and features of the sinus tarsi syndrome. Radiology 1993;186:233-240.
8. Erdman W, Tamburro F, Jayson H, et al: Osteomyelitis: Characteristics and pitfalls of diagnosis with MR imaging. Radiology 1991;180:533-539.
9. Anzilotti K Jr, Schweitzer ME, Hecht P, et al: Effect of foot and ankle MR imaging on clinical decision making. Radiology 1996;201:515-517.

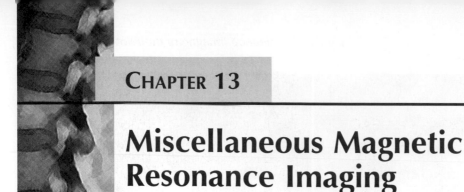

CHAPTER 13

Miscellaneous Magnetic Resonance Imaging

There are several additional areas in which magnetic resonance imaging (MRI) is useful but not well enough developed or of enough widespread use to have an entire chapter devoted to them. Included in this group are MR of the temporomandibular joint (TMJ), wrist, hip, and elbow.

TEMPOROMANDIBULAR JOINT

Diagnostic imaging of the TMJ is performed for so-called internal derangements. I say "so-called" because there is really only one abnormality, for the most part, that makes up the internal derangement: an anteriorly displaced disc. For years disc displacement was diagnosed by arthrography, a painful and somewhat technically demanding study. Some centers replaced arthrography of the TMJ with CT scanning, and now MRI has virtually eliminated all other imaging studies for internal derangements.[1]

Anatomy

The TMJ is a sliding-hinge joint that opens by both hinging and sliding forward (translation). It has a fibrous disc or meniscus that sits on the apex of the condyle and is made up of two thickened portions: the anterior and posterior bands (Fig. 13-1). The thin intermediate zone lies between the anterior and posterior bands. The normal disc has an asymmetric bowtie configuration on sagittal images, with the posterior band larger than the anterior band. The disc is relatively low in signal on all MRI sequences (Fig. 13-2), although some intermediate signal, representing normal hydration, can be seen in the normal posterior band on high-resolution images.

The intermediate zone is an important anatomic landmark because in a normal joint it will always be situated between the two most closely apposed cortical surfaces of the articular eminence of the temporal bone and the condylar head, regardless of whether the mouth is open, closed, or partially open. By using this landmark the disc can be diagnosed as normal in position or anteriorly displaced.

Imaging Technique

Thin section (3 mm), sagittal T1- and T2-weighted images in both a closed and a partially open-mouth position with a small field of view (FOV) and a surface coil are all that are necessary to properly image the TMJ. It is one of the few areas in musculoskeletal imaging in which only one plane of imaging is required.

The partial open-mouth position (mouth open about 10 to 15 mm with gauze or something soft between the teeth to avoid motion) is obtained because occasionally the disc cannot be easily identified on the closed-mouth images because it is crowded into the low-signal glenoid fossa. With partial mouth opening the condyle is not pressing the disc into the glenoid fossa as much, allowing easy identification (see Fig. 13-2). Why not just image only in the partial open-mouth position? Because often the disc reduces to a normal position with minimal mouth opening, and the diagnosis of an anteriorly displaced disc would be missed. If the partial open-mouth images are examined first, the size and shape of the disc can be determined, and then the closed-mouth images can be examined to determine the disc position.

Pathology

In patients with internal derangements of the TMJ, the disc can be found in an anterior position in relation to the condylar head (Fig. 13-3). If the patient is able to open the mouth and the disc

FIGURE 13-1 Schematic of normal temporomandibular joint (TMJ). This drawing shows how the normally positioned TMJ disc lies between the head of the mandibular condyle (C) and the eminence of the temporal bone. The disc has three portions: the anterior band (AB), the larger posterior band (PB), and the thin intermediate zone (IM). The posterior band is over the apex of the condyle in the closed mouth position, as in this example. (Anterior is to the left.) EAC, External auditory canal.

FIGURE 13-2 Normal disc in closed and partial open-mouth positions. *A,* In this T1-weighted sagittal image in the closed-mouth position the disc can be seen as a low-signal, bowtie-shaped structure with the posterior band *(arrow)* superior to the apex of the condyle and the anterior band just anterior to the condylar head. *B,* In the open-mouth position the disc is more easily identified and the posterior band *(arrow)* is noted to have some intermediate signal, indicative of normal hydration. (Anterior is to the left.)

slides back into a normal position, it usually does so with a click or pop that can be painful. This is usually what brings the patient to the dentist or physician. As the process worsens, the disc cannot be returned to the normal position with mouth opening. These patients have some limitation of mouth opening and usually have more severe pain. This has been termed an anteriorly displaced disc without reduction. It has a high incidence of osteoarthritis of the TMJ and often requires surgery to repair or remove the disc.

Because it is easily determined clinically whether the disc reduces (a click or pop is apparent when the disc reduces), I do not spend imaging time trying to determine whether the disc reduces with full mouth opening. Also, reduction of the disc can change from day to day—it may be reducing when the patient is having MRI performed and not when the patient is being examined by his referring doctor. This can lead to some confusion for the referring doctor. In addition, these patients have pain when they open their mouths widely, therefore 10 to 15 minutes in the magnet in a full open-mouth position can be very uncomfortable, which can lead to patient motion and a nondiagnostic study. Because the full open-mouth position is painful and doesn't give the referring physician any information they can't easily determine clinically, I don't obtain such images. The reason I am expounding on this is because most radiologists have recommended imaging the TMJ with the patient's mouth fully open and closed. There appears to be no justification for this.

If the disc is anteriorly displaced and has lost its usual asymmetric bowtie shape (Fig. 13-4), this should be reported. This represents a more severely damaged disc, one that usually cannot be repaired. It has a high association with joint osteoarthritis.

T2-weighted sequences will show fluid in the joint, but offer no additional information on disc position. I usually image both joints simultaneously

FIGURE 13-3   Anteriorly displaced disc. A sagittal T1-weighted image in a partial open-mouth position shows the disc clearly anteriorly displaced with some high signal in the posterior band *(arrow)*. Although it is slightly folded downward, it still has a bowtie shape. (Anterior is to the left.)

FIGURE 13-4   Anteriorly displaced and misshaped disc with degenerative joint disease (DJD). This sagittal T1-weighted image in a patient with advanced TMJ disease shows an anteriorly displaced disc *(arrow)* that has lost its normal bowtie shape and is low in signal throughout, indicative of desiccation. Note the anterior osteophyte on the condyle, indicative of DJD, a common association with advanced TMJ dysfunction.

because we have bilateral coupled coils, but only the symptomatic side needs to be imaged. In the days of arthrography of the TMJ we did not perform bilateral studies routinely. A bilateral study is sometimes useful to get a feel for the anatomy because there is usually some symmetry, but other than that it's not necessary—especially it it's going to cost the patient more than a unilateral study.

WRIST

MRI of the wrist has been slower to develop than that of other joints. Similarly, wrist arthrography has not enjoyed the same popularity as that of the knee or shoulder. Nevertheless, MRI of the wrist has some definite utility. It is useful in evaluating the carpal bones for fractures and avascular necrosis (AVN). It seems to have some use for evaluating the triangular fibrocartilage (TFC) and the intercarpal ligaments.[2]

Imaging Techniques

Thin section (2 to 3 mm) T1- and T2-weighted images in both an axial and a coronal plane are usually used with a dedicated wrist coil or a small surface coil. A small FOV (5 to 8 cm) should be used for maximal resolution. Three-dimensional volumetric images with thin (1 to 2 mm) slices are used in many centers to replace the T2-weighted images. These are especially useful for examining the TFC and the intercarpal ligaments.[3]

Pathology

Triangular Fibrocartilage. The TFC lies between the distal ulna and the carpal bones and is thought to have some shock-absorbing function. It can tear or become detached and cause significant wrist pain and dysfunction. Tears of the TFC can be diagnosed with arthrography or with MRI, although it is somewhat controversial as to the significance of a torn TFC. That is because torn TFCs (and torn intercarpal ligaments, for that matter) are found with a high frequency in older patients who do not have wrist pain or dysfunction. Nevertheless, in a young patient with a painful, torn TFC, most hand surgeons would surgically intervene if conservative care was ineffective. For this reason, imaging may play a role.

The normal TFC is predominantly low signal on all imaging sequences and is seen to be triangular in shape with the base attaching to the ulna and the apex attaching onto the radius (Fig. 13-5). A detached or torn TFC is best seen in the coronal plane with gradient-echo sequences and is usually accompanied by joint fluid in both the distal radioulnar and the proximal carpal joints (Fig. 13-6).

FIGURE 13-5 Normal triangular fibrocartilage (TFC). A coronal gradient-echo three-dimensional volume thin section image of a normal wrist shows the TFC *(arrow)* with its attachment to the radius separated by a thin layer of cartilage.

FIGURE 13-7 Kienböck's malacia. A coronal T1-weighted image shows the lunate *(arrow)* to be devoid of the normal high signal from fatty marrow. This is diagnostic of AVN, called Kienböck's malacia when it occurs in the lunate.

FIGURE 13-6 Torn triangular fibrocartilage (TFC). A coronal gradient-echo three-dimensional volume thin section image of a wrist in a patient with ulnar-sided wrist pain shows the TFC to be torn in its mid-substance *(arrow)*.

Avascular Necrosis. The wrist has several bones that have a propensity to undergo AVN. The lunate is commonly affected and is known as Kienböck's malacia. It is seen as uniform low signal on T1- and T2-weighted images (Fig. 13-7). As is found with AVN in other joints, MRI can be useful in showing AVN when plain films are normal.

The proximal pole of the navicular often undergoes AVN after a fracture. MR can demonstrate the AVN earlier than plain films, allowing earlier treatment. Subtle or occult fractures of the navicular (or any other carpal bone) can be identified with MR. MR should be considered when clinical suspicion of a fracture is high and plain films are negative because a missed fracture of the navicular can lead to AVN. We have found it cost-effective to perform an MR of the wrist to rule out a fracture in a patient with trauma, pain in the snuff box, and a negative plain film, as opposed to casting the patient for a week and having them return for a follow-up x-ray.[4]

Intercarpal Ligaments. The intercarpal ligaments can tear and cause pain and instability in the wrist. They are usually diagnosed arthrographically; however, MRI is beginning to play a role in their evaluation. The scapholunate ligament is the most commonly torn intercarpal ligament. It should be identified at the proximal part of the scapholunate joint in every wrist unless it is torn (Fig. 13-8). The next most common intercarpal ligament to tear is the lunotriquetral ligament, which is found at the proximal portion of the joint. Unfortunately, it is not always visualized, even with excellent images; hence, it is difficult to diagnose a torn lunotriquetral ligament with any certainty.

Further complicating the diagnosis of torn intercarpal ligaments is the fact that they can be torn as a matter of aging and wear and tear without being symptomatic. Hence, diagnosing a torn ligament may have no clinical significance whatsoever. Cadaver studies have reported torn intercarpal ligaments in up to 80% of older people.

FIGURE 13-8 **Scapholunate ligament.** A coronal three-dimensional volume thin section image of a normal wrist shows the appearance of the scapholunate ligament (*arrow*). A normal lunotriquetral ligament (*curved arrow*) also can be seen, although it is not always identified.

Carpal Tunnel Syndrome. The median nerve can become impinged in the carpal tunnel by a variety of processes and result in paresthesia in the hand and fingers. Surgical removal of the offending agent (if any—it is most often idiopathic or caused by overuse of the hands in stressful positions, such as typing) and excision of the flexor retinaculum is usually curative if conservative treatment fails. Although MRI is useful in identifying tumors, ganglia, swollen flexor tendon sheaths, or other masses in the carpal tunnel, many hand surgeons dispute the need for imaging the carpal tunnel because of the ease with which the diagnosis of

carpal tunnel syndrome is made. If surgery is performed, it is easy to inspect the entire carpal tunnel, making preoperative imaging unnecessary.

HIP

The main use of MRI of the hip is to diagnose AVN. It is also used to diagnose hip fractures when plain films are equivocal[5] (hip fractures have been discussed in Chapter 5) and to diagnose a torn acetabular labrum.

AVN can be diagnosed with great sensitivity with MRI. It has a characteristic appearance with involvement of the anterosuperior portion of the femoral head. The area of AVN typically is surrounded by a low-signal serpiginous border (Fig. 13-9). AVN can be diagnosed earlier and more reliably using MRI than with plain films or nuclear medicine.

Acetabular Labrum. The acetabular labrum is analogous to the glenoid labrum of the shoulder. It can tear or detach resulting in a painful, snapping hip. The labrum can be arthroscopically débrided with a good clinical outcome reported by multiple surgeons. For some reason labral debridement has gained popularity on the PGA tour with multiple "big name" golfers having had their labra resected because of hip pain.

The acetabular labrum is best visualized with an MR arthrogram.[6] Imaging should be done with a small FOV and only one hip studied. Bilateral examinations with a large FOV and nonarthrogram studies have an extremely low sensitivity for labral tears. When the labrum tears or detaches, it most commonly is abnormal in the anterosuperior quadrant (Fig. 13-10).

FIGURE 13-9 **Avascular necrosis (AVN) of the femoral head.** A T1-weighted coronal image shows marked low signal in the right femoral head, which indicates advanced hip AVN. The left hip has AVN that shows some high signal surrounded by a low signal serpiginous border. This is characteristic for AVN.

FIGURE 13-10   Torn acetabular labrum. This coronal T1-weighted, fat-suppressed arthrogram of the hip shows fluid between the bony acetabulum and the labrum (*arrow*), indicating a detached labrum.

Idiopathic Transient Osteoporosis of the Hip. Idiopathic transient osteoporosis of the hip is a poorly understood disorder. It is an idiopathic process that begins with a painful hip and no underlying disorder or other findings other than osteoporosis, which is limited to the painful hip. Some believe it is early AVN, whereas others think it is a variant of reflex sympathetic dystrophy. Its appearance on MRI is similar to early AVN[7] in that low signal on T1-weighted images, which is high signal on T2-weighted images, is seen throughout the femoral head and neck (Fig. 13-11). Transient osteoporosis of the hip invariably is self-limited with full resolution. It tends to occur more often in males.

ELBOW

MRI of the elbow has been shown to be useful in diagnosing collateral ligament tears, biceps tendon tears, and for loose bodies. It can show edema in the flexor tendons as they insert on the medial epicondyle and in the extensor tendons on the lateral epicondyle in so-called golfer's and tennis elbow. Bony and cartilaginous abnormalities can also be seen with MRI.

The imaging protocol typically includes axial and coronal T1- and T2-weighted images. Sagittal

A

FIGURE 13-11   Idiopathic transient osteoporosis of the hip. *A,* A plain film of a 40-year-old man with left hip pain shows osteoporosis involving the left hip, with no other abnormalities seen.

Continued

FIGURE 13-11, cont'd   *B,* A T1-weighted (TR, 700; TE, 12) coronal MR examination done at the same time as the plain film shows low signal in the superior portion of the left femoral head. This is a characteristic appearance for AVN, but is a nonspecific finding. Clinically, this patient had no underlying causes for AVN, and he was treated conservatively. *C,* Seven months later, after near total cessation of the hip pain, a repeat MR examination (TR, 600; TE, 20) shows no abnormality in the hip. This is consistent with idiopathic transient osteoporosis of the hip.

A

B

FIGURE 13-12 **Ulnar collateral ligament.** Coronal T1-weighted, fat-suppressed arthrograms of the elbow show the normal ulnar collateral ligament (A) (*arrow*) and one that is torn off of the attachment to the medial epicondyle (B) (*arrow*).

images are optional in some centers; however, we have found them to be useful and routinely obtain a sagittal gradient-echo sequence. MR arthrography is used when a partial tear of the ulnar collateral ligament or loose bodies are clinical considerations.

The ulnar collateral ligament is reliably identified on coronal images. If it is torn, it will show discontinuity and high T2-weighted signal (Fig. 13-12).

REFERENCES

1. Kaplan PA, Helms CA: Current status of temporomandibular joint imaging for the diagnosis of internal derangements. Am J Roentgenol 1989;152:697-705.
2. Kang H, Kindynis P, Brahme S, et al: Triangular fibrocartilage and intercarpal ligaments of the wrist: MR imaging. Cadaveric study with gross pathologic and histologic correlation. Radiology 1991;181:401-404.
3. Totterman S, Miller R, Wasserman B, et al: Intrinsic and extrinsic carpal ligaments: Evaluation by three-dimensional Fourier transform MR imaging. Am J Roentgenol 1993;160:117-123.
4. Dorsay TA, Major NM, Helms CA: Cost-effectiveness of immediate MR imaging versus traditional follow-up for revealing radiographically occult scaphoid fractures. AJR Am J Roentgenol 2001;177:1257-1263.
5. Rizzo P, Gould E, Lyden J, Asnis S: Diagnosis of occult fractures about the hip. MRI compared with bone-scanning. J Bone Joint Surg 1993;75-A:395-401.
6. Petersilge CA: MR arthrography for evaluation of the acetabular labrum. Skeletal Radiol 2001;30:423-430.
7. Takatori Y, Kokubo T, Ninomiya S, et al: Transient osteoporosis of the hip. Magnetic resonance imaging. Clin Orthop Relat Res 1991;271:190-194.

Index